VARICOSE VEINS

Foods, Supplements & Herbs

Isabel M. Rivero

COPYRIGHT & CREDITS

VARICOSE VEINS. Foods, Supplements & Herbs.
Copyright ©2018, 2024 *by* Isabel M. Rivero
All rights reserved

Photographs by Buntysmum and Marikusa via Pixabay

This book provides general information and is not a substitute for professional medical advice. Neither the publisher nor the author shall be held liable for any damages of any kind arising from the use of this content. Readers assume full responsibility for their decisions, actions, and outcomes.

This book is intended as a reference only and should never be used as a medical manual. Its purpose is to help readers make informed decisions about their health. It is not intended to replace any treatment prescribed by a doctor.

Original title: *VARICES. Alimentos y Plantas Medicinales* © 2018, Isabel M. Rivero. All Rights Reserved
© 2024 translated by Laura Mendoza & Sara I. Afonso

Prologue: A Guide to Wellness

Dear Readers,

Welcome to this journey toward better health! Since I began sharing my knowledge and experience, my primary motivation has been to make a positive contribution to your lives. That's why, through these pages, I aim to offer valuable information and practical resources that can genuinely help you feel better.

In this book, every piece of advice and remedy has been thoughtfully chosen for its proven effectiveness and practicality in everyday life. You will discover not only medicinal plants, supplements, and accessible foods but also detailed medical insights into this health concern, along with additional tips and answers to the most frequently asked questions–providing you with a practical, comprehensive, and trustworthy guide.

My goal is for this work to be your valuable and practical companion–a resource where you can find tangible tools to support you on your journey toward a healthier, more fulfilling life. Knowing that this work has a positive impact brings me great joy and motivates me to keep going. While writing requires effort, time, and perseverance, the knowledge that my books make a meaningful difference in your lives is my greatest reward.

Because your experiences are my greatest source of inspiration, I would love for you to write to me and share your progress. Feel free to share your progress by writing directly to me at **isabelmriveror@gmail.com**. Your stories inspire me and truly make my efforts worthwhile.

I sincerely hope this practical guide becomes your indispensable pillar on your journey to better health and well-being. Thank you for allowing me to be part of your life.

With love,

Isabel

INTRODUCTION

On our journey toward optimal health, it's essential to understand that no "miracle" remedy–whether it's a medication, herb, supplement, or food–can fully address an illness on its own. Similarly, focusing solely on alleviating symptoms without addressing the underlying "cause" increases the risk of relapse. Treating the root of the problem, however, gradually reduces symptoms and promotes true and lasting recovery.

You may have noticed that, at times, medications don't work as expected. This happens because regaining health requires a holistic treatment approach that addresses the actual cause of the problem at its root. In addition to effective treatments, this approach should include changes in diet, sleep quality, stress management, and overall lifestyle habits.

With this book, we will explore a holistic approach to health. In the first chapter, you'll find key information to help you understand the main causes of this disease, along with its symptoms, types, warning signs, common complications, helpful advice, and the essential medical tests needed for an accurate diagnosis. In the following chapters, we'll dive into strategies to support recovery, including dietary guidance, daily menus, and natural approaches such as supplements and herbal remedies for gradual improvement.

While you can select your preferred remedies independently, the chapter **"Suggested Practical Plan"** will serve as your primary guide. This section provides a comprehensive approach, addressing all essential aspects of recovery. From there, you'll gain access to the other chapters and apply the recommendations most suited to your unique situation.

It's important to emphasize that the benefits of the recommendations provided in this book are grounded in scientific evidence, rather than personal opinions. At the end, you'll find references and studies supporting each remedy, ensuring you feel confident and secure when applying them.

VARICOSE VEINS

Varicose veins are a common medical condition that affects a significant number of people. They manifest as dilated and elongated superficial veins, particularly in the legs. This condition occurs when venous valves, responsible for preventing blood from flowing backward, become weakened or damaged. As a result, proper blood circulation is disrupted, leading to pooling and accumulation that eventually impacts the affected veins.

The veins in the legs are specifically tasked with returning blood to the heart, working continuously against gravity. To achieve this, they utilize one-way valves that direct blood upward and prevent it from flowing back down. When these valves fail to function properly, blood tends to accumulate, increasing venous pressure and contributing to the development of varicose veins.

The consequences of varicose veins extend beyond aesthetics. The affected veins, which become visibly swollen and often turn bluish or purplish, can cause emotional discomfort for those who experience them. Beyond their appearance, they are frequently accompanied by symptoms such as heaviness, swelling, pain, itching, cramps, and heightened sensitivity. These symptoms can significantly impact quality of life and often worsen after prolonged periods of standing or sitting.

The root cause of varicose veins is related to the deterioration of venous valves, resulting in backward blood flow and increased pressure on the vein walls. Over time, this persistent pressure weakens and dilates the veins, leading to varicose formations that worsen as the condition progresses.

A crucial factor in their development is venous hypertension, which inhibits the return of blood to the heart due to malfunctioning valves or obstructions. This heightened pressure compromises the structural integrity of the veins, making them more fragile and prone to abnormal dilation. Additionally, the quality of the connective tissue in venous walls plays a vital role, as the degeneration of components like collagen and elastin can cause the veins to lose their flexibility and strength. This degeneration may be accelerated by factors such as genetics, aging, hormonal changes, or certain medical conditions, including those associated with pregnancy.

Lifestyle choices also significantly influence the development of varicose veins. Prolonged periods of sitting or standing can slow venous return, increase venous pressure, and encourage blood pooling. A sedentary lifestyle combined with poor posture further exacerbates the issue.

For women, hormonal changes are a key determinant in the development of varicose veins. Hormones like estrogen can weaken venous walls, making them more susceptible to dilation. These effects are further intensified during pregnancy due to increased blood volume and the additional pressure exerted by the growing uterus. Consequently, women are at a higher risk of developing varicose veins, particularly during pregnancy.

Inflammation also plays a critical role in the development and progression of varicose veins. The prolonged accumulation of blood in the veins triggers an inflammatory response, further weakening the venous walls and accelerating their degeneration over time.

In summary, varicose veins result from the interplay of multiple factors: valvular insufficiency, venous hypertension, connective tissue degeneration, circulatory deficiencies, hormonal influences, and chronic inflammatory responses. Combined with genetic predisposition, these factors contribute to the progression of the condition. Understanding these mechanisms is essential to improve both diagnosis and treatment.

Although varicose veins are typically not life-threatening,

they can cause substantial discomfort that adversely affects the physical and emotional well-being of those affected. Common symptoms such as pain, heaviness, itching, and cramps can become more severe following prolonged inactivity. Their impact also extends beyond physical discomfort; many people experience diminished self-confidence due to the visible appearance of their legs, which can negatively affect their self-esteem.

That said, it's important to remember that you are not alone in facing this condition—and there are solutions that can make a significant difference. Even in advanced cases, proper management of varicose veins can provide relief from symptoms, help prevent complications, and restore a higher quality of life. This book is here to guide you with detailed information, practical advice, and natural remedies to help you regain control of your well-being. Stay strong! Knowledge is the first step toward taking care of yourself and feeling better.

This revised version ensures the language flows smoothly and maintains clarity while aligning with American English grammar and style.

Types of Varicose Veins

Varicose veins are not all the same, as they can present in various forms depending on their characteristics and the areas of the body where they develop. Below, you'll find an overview of the main types of varicose veins, helping you better understand their unique features and how they may impact your overall well-being.

- **Varicose veins of the lower extremities**: This is the most common type of varicose veins and mainly affects the legs. These veins are characterized by dilated superficial veins, which become tortuous and prominent. They may be blue or purple and often appear as bulges or cords under the skin. Symptoms may include pain, swelling, itching, heaviness, and muscle cramps.

- **Esophageal varices**: Esophageal varices are dilated veins in the esophagus, the tube that connects the mouth to the stomach. They usually result from underlying liver disease, such as cirrhosis, which causes increased pressure in the veins of the portal system. Esophageal varices can be dangerous, as they can cause severe bleeding. Properly monitoring and treating liver disease is essential to prevent its occurrence.

• **Pelvic varicose veins**: These are dilated veins in the pelvic region, which includes the uterus, ovaries, and pelvis. They can be caused by venous insufficiency in the pelvic veins, which leads to blood pooling and dilation. While they may be asymptomatic in some cases, they can cause chronic pelvic pain, pain during sexual intercourse, a feeling of pressure in the pelvis, and alterations in the menstrual cycle.

• **Vulvar varicose veins**: These are dilated veins in women's external genital region, specifically in the labia majora and labia minora. They may be caused by venous insufficiency in the pelvic area, leading to an accumulation of blood in the vulvar veins. These veins can be painful and cause discomfort during pregnancy, childbirth, and the menstrual cycle.

• **Hemorrhoidal varicose veins**: These are dilated veins in the area of the anus and rectum. They are common and can be caused by increased pressure in the hemorrhoidal veins, such as chronic constipation, pregnancy, or heavy lifting. Symptoms may include pain, itching, bleeding, and a burning sensation.

• **Facial varicose veins**: Also known as spider veins or telangiectasias, these are dilated veins that appear on the face, especially on the cheeks, nose, and forehead. They are small and appear as red or blue lines on the skin. Although usually cosmetic and not causing symptoms, some people may experience redness, tenderness, or burning in the affected areas.

• **Reticular varicose veins**: These are larger than spider veins but smaller than varicose veins of the lower extremities. They appear as a net or mesh on the skin and may be blue-green or reddish. Unlike varicose veins of the legs, reticular varicose veins usually do not cause significant pain or discomfort, but they can be a cosmetic concern for some people.

• **Pelvic varicose veins**: Also known as deep pelvic varicose veins, these are dilated veins found in the pelvic area. They are more common in women and may be associated with pregnancy, hormonal changes, or pressure exerted on the veins due to the position of the uterus. Pelvic varicose veins can cause chronic pelvic pain and discomfort during intercourse and may, in some cases, cause infertility.

• **Congenital varicose veins**: Some people are born with varicose veins, known as congenital varicose veins. These may be the result of a malformation in the veins from birth. Although less common than acquired varicose veins, they can be more severe and require more aggressive treatment.

• **Varicose veins secondary to medical conditions**: Certain medical conditions may increase the risk of developing varicose veins. For instance, heart failure, Cockett's syndrome (compression of the iliac vein by the iliac artery), deep vein thrombosis, and May-Thurner syndrome (compression of the left iliac vein by the right iliac artery) can lead to the development of varicose veins due to altered blood flow.

• **Spinal varicose veins**: These are dilated veins found in the spinal cord. This type is rare and may be caused by a congenital malformation or spinal cord injury. Spinal varicose veins can compress nerves and cause symptoms such as back pain, muscle weakness, loss of sensation, and even problems with bladder or bowel control.

• **Visceral varices**: These are dilated veins found in internal organs, such as the liver, spleen, or intestines. They may be the result of severe liver disease, such as cirrhosis, which causes increased pressure in the veins of the portal system. Visceral varices can be dangerous, as they can bleed and cause serious complications, such as internal bleeding.

• **Labial varicose veins**: These are dilated veins found in the lips and mouth. Although rare, they may result from venous insufficiency in the blood vessels of the lips. Labial varicose veins can be painful and cause discomfort when speaking, eating, or even smiling.

If you're worried about varicose veins or experiencing related discomfort, don't hesitate to consult a vein specialist. These experts are trained to provide a thorough evaluation, including a detailed physical examination, a review of your medical history, and specialized diagnostic tests if needed. Taking this step could make a significant difference in your health and well-being!

Symptoms

Varicose veins can lead to a variety of symptoms, with the intensity and level of discomfort differing from one person to another.

• **Visible appearance**: One of the most obvious symptoms of varicose veins is the presence of dilated and tortuous veins that are visible to the naked eye. These veins may be dark blue or purple and protrude above the skin's surface. Truncal varicose veins are usually the largest and most prominent, while reticular varicose veins and spider veins (telangiectasias) are smaller and look like branching or spider-like webs.

• **Feeling of heaviness or tiredness in the legs**: Many people with varicose veins experience a sense of heaviness or fatigue, especially after standing or sitting for long periods. This is because the accumulation of blood in the affected veins puts extra pressure on the legs, making venous return difficult and causing fatigue or heaviness.

• **Pain or discomfort**: Some people may experience pain or discomfort in their legs due to varicose veins. The pain can range from a burning or stinging sensation to muscle cramps or tenderness in the affected areas. It may worsen when standing or walking for long periods and improve when elevating the legs or resting.

• **Swelling**: The accumulation of blood and pressure in the veins affected by varicose veins can cause swelling in the legs and ankles. This swelling, known as edema, is usually more pronounced at the end of the day and may improve with rest and leg elevation.

• **Night cramps**: Some people with varicose veins may experience muscle cramps in their legs at night. These cramps are often painful and may awaken the person from sleep. Night cramps are thought to be related to poor blood circulation and the accumulation of waste products in the leg muscles.

• **Skin changes**: In more advanced cases of varicose veins, skin changes may occur on the legs. These changes may include dryness, itching, redness, or skin discoloration. Additionally, the skin around varicose veins may become thinner and more fragile, increasing the risk of developing varicose ulcers.

• **Varicose ulcers**: Varicose ulcers are open wounds that form on the skin, usually on the lower leg or around the ankle. These ulcers are the result of blood stagnation in the veins affected by varicose veins, leading to a lack of oxygen and nutrients in the skin. Varicose ulcers can be painful, can become infected, and require specialized medical care for treatment and healing.

• **Itchy and tender skin**: Some people with varicose veins may experience itchy skin on the affected legs. This is due to the accumulation of blood and the extra pressure on the veins, which can cause skin irritation. Additionally, the skin around varicose veins may become more sensitive to touch and may ache or feel sore.

• **Changes in skin temperature**: Varicose veins can affect blood circulation in the legs, which can cause changes in skin temperature. Some people may notice that the skin on the legs affected by varicose veins feels cooler or warmer than the rest of the body.

- **Changes in nail appearance**: In more advanced cases of varicose veins, poor blood circulation can affect the supply of nutrients and oxygen to the toenails, resulting in changes in the appearance of the nails, such as thickening, discoloration, or brittleness.

- **Tingling sensation or numbness**: Some people may experience tingling sensations or numbness in the legs due to varicose veins. This may be due to the extra pressure the enlarged veins exert on nearby nerves.

- **Aggravation of symptoms during pregnancy**: Hormones and increased blood volume during pregnancy can increase the likelihood of developing varicose veins or worsen existing symptoms. Many pregnant women may experience swelling, pain, or heaviness in their legs due to varicose veins.

- **Changes in skin texture**: In advanced cases of varicose veins, the accumulation of blood and poor circulation can affect the nutrition and oxygenation of the skin. This can result in changes in skin texture, such as dryness, flaking, or hardening. The skin may also become more prone to injury and may take longer to heal.

- **Appearance of varicose veins in other areas of the body**: Although varicose veins are most common in the legs, they can also develop in other areas of the body, such as the arms, abdomen, or pelvic region. These varicose veins may present symptoms similar to those in the legs, such as swelling, pain, or changes in the appearance of the skin.

- **Sensitivity to hot or cold weather**: Some people with varicose veins may experience sensitivity to cold or hot weather in the affected legs. This is due to altered blood circulation and the body's response to temperature changes.

- **Tingling sensation or sensitivity to touch**: The pressure exerted by the dilated veins on nearby nerves may cause some people to experience tingling, tenderness, or even pain when touching or pressing on the affected areas.

• **Changes in the appearance of the legs when standing**: Some people may notice that varicose veins become more prominent or swell even more when standing for long periods. This is due to the increased pressure on the veins and the difficulty of blood flowing correctly.

• **Changes in the appearance of the legs after exercise**: After exercise or intense physical activity, varicose veins may become more visible or cause more discomfort in some people. This is due to increased blood flow and increased pressure on the veins during physical activity.

It is crucial to understand that the symptoms of varicose veins can differ significantly from one person to another. While some individuals may experience mild and occasional discomfort, others may endure more severe and persistent symptoms. Moreover, if left untreated, these symptoms can progressively worsen over time.

If you notice any of these signs or have concerns about varicose veins, don't hesitate to consult a vein specialist. Their expertise ensures that you receive an accurate and personalized diagnosis.

Remember, seeking timely treatment not only helps relieve symptoms but also improves circulation and prevents serious complications like ulcers or deep vein thrombosis. Taking action early is essential for your health and overall well-being!

Causes

Varicose veins develop due to a combination of genetic and environmental factors that disrupt the normal functioning of veins. The main causes include:

• **Venous insufficiency**: This is one of the most common causes of varicose veins. Venous insufficiency occurs when the valves in the veins of the legs do not function properly. These valves are responsible for helping blood flow in only one direction, toward the heart. When the valves do not close properly, blood can back up and pool in the veins, resulting in their dilation and the formation of varicose veins.

• **Genetics**: Genetic predisposition also plays an essential role in the development of varicose veins. If you have close relatives, such as parents or siblings, who have had varicose veins, you are more likely to develop them as well. This is because the structure and function of veins can be passed down from generation to generation.

• **Age**: Our veins may lose elasticity and weaken their walls as we age, causing them to dilate and become varicose. Our venous valves may also deteriorate, contributing to venous insufficiency.

• **Gender**: Women are more likely to develop varicose veins compared to men. This is partly due to hormonal changes that occur during pregnancy, menstruation, and menopause, which can weaken vein walls and affect valve function. In addition, the use of hormonal contraceptives may increase the risk of developing varicose veins.

• **Pregnancy**: During pregnancy, the body experiences hormonal changes and an increase in blood volume to support the growing fetus. These changes can put additional pressure on the veins in the legs and make venous return more difficult. As a result, many pregnant women develop varicose veins or experience a worsening of existing symptoms.

• **Obesity**: Excess body weight can put additional pressure on leg veins, which hinders proper blood flow. In addition, obesity may be associated with a sedentary lifestyle and poor circulation, which increases the risk of developing varicose veins.

• **Sedentary lifestyle**: Sitting or standing for long periods without moving can hinder proper blood flow and increase the risk of developing varicose veins. A sedentary lifestyle can also contribute to weight gain and obesity, further exacerbating the problem.

- **Injuries or trauma to the legs**: Injuries or trauma to the legs can damage veins and valves, hindering proper blood flow and contributing to the development of varicose veins.

- **Other risk factors**: Besides the causes mentioned above, other risk factors can increase the likelihood of developing varicose veins. These include wearing tight clothing, prolonged use of high heels, prolonged exposure to heat (such as hot baths or saunas), and specific jobs that involve standing or sitting for long periods.

- **High blood pressure**: High blood pressure can put additional pressure on the veins and hinder proper blood flow, which increases the risk of developing varicose veins.

- **Liver disease**: Some liver diseases, such as liver cirrhosis, can affect blood flow and vein function, increasing the risk of developing varicose veins.

- **Chronic constipation**: Chronic constipation can increase abdominal pressure, hinder proper blood flow, and contribute to the development of varicose veins.

- **Prolonged sun exposure**: Prolonged sun exposure can weaken vein walls and affect valve function, increasing the risk of developing varicose veins.

- **Smoking**: Smoking can damage veins and affect blood circulation, which increases the risk of developing varicose veins.

- **Medications**: Some drugs, such as oral contraceptives and hormone treatments, can increase the risk of developing varicose veins. Additionally, certain medications used to treat conditions such as cancer or high blood pressure can affect blood circulation and contribute to the development of varicose veins.

- **History of blood clots**: People who have had blood clots in their veins (deep vein thrombosis) are at an increased risk of developing varicose veins. Clots can damage veins and affect blood circulation, leading to varicose veins.

• **Intense physical activity or heavy lifting**: Regularly performing high-impact physical activities or lifting heavy objects can put additional pressure on the veins and contribute to the development of varicose veins.

• **Connective tissue diseases**: Some connective tissue diseases, such as Ehlers-Danlos syndrome or systemic lupus erythematosus, can weaken vein walls and increase the risk of developing varicose veins.

• **Excess stress**: Chronic stress can negatively affect blood circulation and contribute to the development of varicose veins. Additionally, stress can lead to unhealthy habits, such as poor diet or lack of exercise, which can also increase the risk of varicose veins.

• **Hormonal changes**: In addition to hormonal changes associated with pregnancy, menstruation, and menopause, other hormonal changes, such as those that occur during puberty, can affect vein health and increase the risk of developing varicose veins.

• **Exposure to toxic chemicals**: Certain harmful substances, such as those found in pesticides or cleaning products, can damage veins and contribute to the development of varicose veins.

It is important to understand that varicose veins are typically caused by a combination of factors, with each individual having unique underlying causes. While certain factors, such as genetics, are beyond control, others can be managed or modified.

Possible Complications

This section is designed to provide clear guidance and highlight potential risks, with a strong emphasis on prevention. By doing so, you can take proactive steps to safeguard your well-being and minimize the likelihood of complications.

Varicose veins are not just a cosmetic concern; they can also lead to complications that affect both your overall health and quality of life. These complications can range from mild discomfort to more serious medical conditions. Below is a comprehensive overview of the primary complications associated with varicose veins.

- **Venous ulcers**: Varicose veins can increase the risk of developing venous ulcers and open sores on the skin that can be painful and difficult to heal. These ulcers typically form on the lower leg, near the ankle, and result from blood pooling in the affected veins and poor circulation. Venous ulcers can be painful, become infected, and may require specialized medical care for treatment.

- **Deep vein thrombosis (DVT)**: Deep vein thrombosis is a condition in which a blood clot forms in a deep vein, usually in the leg. Varicose veins can increase the risk of developing DVT, as dilated and damaged veins can encourage blood clots to form. DVT can be a severe and life-threatening condition if a clot breaks loose and travels to the lungs, causing a pulmonary embolism.

- **Phlebitis**: Phlebitis is inflammation of a vein and can occur in varicose veins. The presence of varicose veins can increase the risk of developing phlebitis, as dilated and damaged veins can become irritated and inflamed. Phlebitis can cause pain, redness, and a feeling of warmth in the affected area. In some cases, phlebitis can lead to the formation of blood clots and more severe complications.

- **Hemorrhages**: In rare cases, varicose veins can rupture and cause bleeding. This can occur if the vein walls become weak enough to rupture or if excessive pressure is applied to them due to trauma or injury. Varicose vein bleeding can be severe and require immediate medical attention.

- **Hyperpigmentation and skin changes**: Chronic varicose veins can cause skin changes such as hyperpigmentation (dark spots), venous eczema (inflammation of the skin), dermatitis, or even ulcers. These skin changes can be uncomfortable and affect a person's quality of life.

• **Pelvic congestion syndrome**: In some women, varicose veins can also develop in the pelvic region, known as pelvic congestion syndrome. This can cause chronic pelvic pain, discomfort during intercourse, and other symptoms related to venous congestion in the pelvis.

• **Bleeding**: Varicose veins can be prone to bleeding, especially if the affected area is traumatized or injured. Although bleeding from varicose veins is not common, it can be challenging to control and requires urgent medical attention.

• **Infections**: Varicose veins can increase the risk of developing vein infections, known as infectious phlebitis. This can occur if varicose veins become damaged or rupture, allowing bacteria to enter the veins. Vein infections can be severe and require treatment with antibiotics.

• **Chronic venous insufficiency**: Varicose veins are a manifestation of chronic venous insufficiency, a condition in which the veins cannot efficiently pump blood back to the heart. As varicose veins worsen, there can be increased pooling of blood in the veins and increased pressure in the lower extremities. This can lead to symptoms such as heaviness, pain, swelling, and tiredness in the legs.

• **Post-thrombotic syndrome**: If deep vein thrombosis develops in varicose veins, damage to the venous valves and vein walls can occur. This can result in a condition known as post-thrombotic syndrome, which is characterized by chronic pain, swelling, skin discoloration, changes, and ulcers in the affected area.

• **Aesthetic and emotional problems**: Varicose veins can have a negative impact on the aesthetic appearance of the legs, which can affect a person's self-esteem and confidence. Additionally, some people may experience anxiety or depression related to varicose veins and their associated symptoms.

• **Varicorragia**: Varicorragia refers to sudden, profuse bleeding from a varicose vein. It can occur when a varicose vein ruptures or is damaged due to pressure exerted on it. Varicorragia can be an alarming event and may require emergency medical attention to stop the bleeding.

• **Skin ulcers**: Advanced varicose veins can lead to venous ulcers, which are open, hard-to-heal wounds on the skin, usually on the lower leg or ankle. These ulcers can be painful and can take a long time to heal, sometimes even months or years. They require proper and constant medical care to prevent infection and promote healing.

• **Nerve compression syndrome**: Advanced varicose veins can put pressure on nearby nerves, leading to nerve compression syndrome. This can cause pain, numbness, tingling, or weakness in the legs. Nerve compression syndrome can affect quality of life and require medical treatment.

• **Erythema nodosum**: Erythema nodosum is an inflammatory skin reaction that can occur in people with advanced varicose veins. It manifests as painful, red bumps on the skin, usually on the legs. Erythema nodosum can be uncomfortable and requires medical attention to relieve symptoms and treat the underlying cause.

• **Circulation problems**: Varicose veins can adversely affect blood circulation in the legs. The accumulation of blood in the dilated veins can hinder blood flow back to the heart, resulting in swelling, fatigue, cramping, and heaviness in the legs. Additionally, poor circulation can increase the risk of developing blood clots.

• **Complications during pregnancy**: Varicose veins are common due to hormonal changes and increased blood volume. In some women, they may worsen during pregnancy, leading to complications such as deep vein thrombosis and increased leg discomfort. Pregnant women must follow medical recommendations and take measures to prevent and control varicose veins during this period.

Symptom Relief and Prevention

Relieving symptoms and preventing varicose veins are essential for maintaining vascular health and avoiding potential complications. Below are a series of key recommendations to promote the well-being of your veins and prevent future issues.

- **Maintain an active lifestyle**: Regular physical activity is essential to maintain good blood circulation and strengthen leg muscles. Engage in exercises that stimulate your leg muscles, such as walking, running, swimming, or cycling. Avoid being sedentary for long periods, and if you have a job that requires prolonged standing or sitting, try to take regular breaks to move and stretch.

- **Control your weight**: Maintaining a healthy weight is essential to reduce pressure on leg veins. Excess weight and obesity can increase the risk of developing varicose veins. If you are overweight, working to reduce your weight can help alleviate symptoms and prevent varicose veins.

- **Elevate your legs**: Elevating your legs above the level of your heart can help reduce blood pooling in your veins and relieve the symptoms of varicose veins. Do this several times a day for 15-20 minutes, especially after prolonged periods of standing or sitting.

- **Avoid tight clothing**: Wearing tight clothing, such as tight pants or excessive compression stockings, can impede blood flow and worsen varicose vein symptoms. Opt for loose-fitting, comfortable clothing that does not compress the legs.

- **Maintain good vascular hygiene**: Take care of your legs by keeping them clean and hydrated. Avoid prolonged exposure to the sun and heat, as this can dilate the veins. Use moisturizing creams and avoid products containing skin-irritating ingredients.

- **Avoid constipation**: Constipation can increase pressure in the abdomen and make it difficult for blood to flow back from the legs. To maintain a healthy digestive system and prevent constipation, maintain a fiber-rich diet and drink enough water.

- **Wear compression stockings**: Compression stockings can help relieve the symptoms of varicose veins. They apply gradual pressure to the legs, which helps improve blood flow and reduce swelling. Consult a physician for advice on the proper type and pressure of compression stockings.

- **Avoid smoking**: Smoking damages blood vessels and affects circulation. Quitting smoking can significantly improve vascular health and reduce the risk of developing varicose veins.

- **Manage hormonal changes**: If you are pregnant or in menopause, talk to your doctor about how to manage hormonal changes to minimize the impact on your veins. They may recommend hormone therapies or specific preventive measures.

- **Have regular medical check-ups**: If you have a family history of varicose veins or have symptoms, it is essential to have regular medical check-ups with a vascular disease specialist.

- **Avoid crossing your legs**: Crossing your legs can hinder blood flow and increase pressure in your legs' veins. Try to keep your legs in a neutral position and avoid crossing them when sitting.

- **Raise the feet of the bed**: Slightly elevate the feet of your bed, about 10 to 15 centimeters, to help improve circulation while you sleep.

- **Control blood pressure**: High blood pressure can increase the risk of developing varicose veins. Keep your blood pressure under control through a healthy diet, regular exercise, stress reduction, and, if necessary, medications prescribed by a physician.

- **Avoid prolonged use of high heels**: Frequent use of high heels can hinder blood flow in the legs. Try alternating between heels and flats to give your legs a break and improve circulation.

• **Maintain a healthy diet**: A balanced, nutrient-rich diet can help maintain vascular health. Include foods rich in fiber, fruits, and vegetables, as well as lean proteins and healthy fats. Avoid excess salt, which can contribute to fluid retention and worsen leg swelling.

• **Avoid excessive exposure to heat**: Heat dilates the veins and can worsen the symptoms of varicose veins. Avoid prolonged hot baths and saunas and direct sun exposure during the hottest part of the day.

• **Manage stress**: Chronic stress can affect vascular health and worsen varicose vein symptoms. Look for ways to reduce stress in your life, such as practicing relaxation techniques, meditation, yoga, or activities that please you.

• **Massage your legs**: Gentle leg massages can help stimulate blood circulation and relieve symptoms of varicose veins. Apply upward circular motions with a moisturizing cream or oil to help reduce swelling and improve blood flow.

• **Apply cold compresses**: Cold compresses can help relieve swelling and discomfort associated with varicose veins. Apply a cold compress or ice pack wrapped in a cloth to the affected areas for a few minutes several times a day.

• **Always end your bath with a splash of cold water on your legs**.

• **Do "gymnastics" for the veins**. These are easy exercises that activate blood flow. The best ones are the following:

   - Walk.
   - Walk alternately on tiptoe and on heels.
   - Lie on your back and "pedal" in the air.
   - Shrink and stretch your toes.
   - Roll the feet from the heels to the toes and back.
   - Grasp and lift a cloth or light object with the toes.

- Rest the front of your feet on a step. Raise and lower your heels.
- Sitting on a chair, support your heels and raise your toes, or vice versa.

• **Andullation therapy**: This therapy is highly recommended for the treatment of varicose veins due to its effects on blood circulation. This biophysical therapy also stimulates deep metabolism, which allows a better supply of nutrients and oxygen to the body tissues. In addition, it can stop the progression of varicose veins and prevent their worsening. If you are interested in trying andullation, you can search the internet for the word "andullation" along with the country you live in to find the corresponding website. From there, you can request a free, no-obligation trial of this therapy.

Additional Tips

Adopting healthy and practical habits can make a significant difference in caring for your veins and alleviating symptoms. In this section, you'll find complementary recommendations covering topics such as hydration, nutrition, specific therapies, and daily activities. These strategies will not only help improve the health of your blood vessels but also enhance your overall well-being. Discover how you can put them into practice!

• **Adequate hydration**: Maintaining proper hydration is crucial for preserving the elasticity of blood vessels and facilitating blood flow. Drink enough water throughout the day to stay well hydrated.

• **Healthy eating**: A balanced diet of fruits, vegetables, whole grains, and lean proteins can support blood vessel health. Additionally, include foods high in vitamin C, such as citrus fruits, strawberries, and peppers, as this vitamin is essential for vascular health.

• **Avoid excessive salt intake**: Consuming too much salt can lead to fluid retention and exacerbate the swelling associated with varicose veins. Limit your intake of processed foods and avoid adding extra salt to your meals.

• **Compression therapy**: Besides compression stockings, other options include elastic bandages or intermittent pneumatic compression devices.

• **Avoid passive smoking**: In addition to avoiding smoking, it is vital to minimize exposure to secondhand smoke. Passive smoking can negatively impact blood vessel health and overall circulation.

• **Eat foods rich in antioxidants**: Antioxidants, such as vitamins A, C, and E, help protect blood vessels from oxidative damage. Include foods like carrots, oranges, spinach, nuts, and olive oil in your diet to ensure a good intake of antioxidants.

• **Avoid activities that put excessive pressure on the legs**: Some intense activities, such as weightlifting or high-impact exercise, can put undue pressure on the legs and worsen varicose veins. Opt for low-impact activities like walking, swimming, or cycling.

• **Topical ointments** may help reduce discomfort.

• **Hydrotherapy**, especially the combination of cold and heat, is highly effective in activating circulation and relieving itching, burning, and pain in the legs.

• If possible, **walk along the seashore** to combine physical activity with the refreshing effects of the water.

• Before going to bed, perform **pedaling movements** to promote venous return during sleep.

• **Green clay**: Mix green clay with water to create a consistent mixture. Apply it to the affected areas and allow it to dry completely. Then rinse with warm or cold water and use a neutral soap.

Diagnostic Medical Tests

Diagnostic medical tests play an essential role in evaluating and diagnosing venous conditions. These tools allow healthcare professionals to assess the state of the veins, identify potential complications, and determine the most appropriate treatment tailored to each case. Below is an overview of some of the most commonly used diagnostic tests.

- **Physical exam:** The first step in diagnosing varicose veins is a physical examination by a vein specialist, such as a phlebologist or vascular surgeon. During the examination, the physician will visually assess the legs for dilated and twisted veins, and the veins may also be palpated to determine their size, texture, and tenderness.

- **Medical history and symptoms:** The doctor will gather information about your symptoms, such as pain, heaviness, cramping, or leg swelling. It is also essential to inform the doctor of any family history of varicose veins or circulation problems.

- **Doppler ultrasound:** Doppler ultrasound is a non-invasive and widely used test for diagnosing varicose veins. It uses high-frequency sound waves to produce real-time images of the veins and evaluate their blood flow. Doppler allows the physician to view the veins in detail and determine if abnormal or backward blood flow is in the affected veins.

- **Duplex ultrasound:** Duplex ultrasound combines conventional ultrasound with blood flow analysis using the Doppler technique. This test provides real-time images of veins and blood flow, allowing a more detailed evaluation of varicose veins and their complications, such as the presence of blood clots or valvular insufficiency.

- **Phlebography:** Phlebography is an invasive test that is rarely used today but may be necessary in complex cases or when other tests are inconclusive. It involves injecting a contrast dye into the veins and taking X-rays to visualize the veins and any abnormalities. Phlebography provides a more detailed picture of the venous system and can help determine the best treatment approach.

• **Photoplethysmography**: Photoplethysmography uses light sensors to measure changes in blood volume in the legs. It provides information about venous function and pressure, which can help assess the severity of varicose veins and blood flow in the legs.

• **Magnetic Resonance Venography (MRV)** is a noninvasive imaging technique that uses magnetic fields and radio waves to create detailed images of the venous system. It is especially useful for evaluating deep veins and detecting blockages or abnormalities in blood flow. MRV can provide accurate information about venous anatomy and help plan treatments such as sclerotherapy or surgery.

• **Thermography**: Thermography uses a thermal camera to measure the temperature of the skin on the legs. Varicose veins can cause changes in skin temperature, which this test can detect. Thermography can provide additional information about blood flow and venous function, especially in cases of asymptomatic varicose veins.

• **Ankle-brachial index (ABI)**: The ABI test evaluates arterial circulation in the legs. It measures blood pressure in the arms and ankles and compares the results. If blood pressure in the ankles decreases significantly compared to that in the arms, this may indicate poor blood circulation in the legs, which could be a risk factor for developing varicose veins.

• **Coagulation studies**: In some cases, blood coagulation tests may be performed to rule out coagulation disorders that may increase the risk of developing varicose veins or associated complications, such as deep vein thrombosis.

It is essential to note that the choice of diagnostic tests will depend on your specific case and what your doctor determines to be necessary. Not all the tests mentioned are used in every case of varicose veins, as each individual and their symptoms are unique. Your doctor may combine multiple tests to achieve a clearer and more comprehensive diagnosis. This step is crucial to fully understand your condition and provide you with the most appropriate treatment.

Warning Signs

While varicose veins are often merely a cosmetic concern, they can sometimes indicate a more serious underlying issue. That's why I want to help you identify potential warning signs, enabling you to detect any complications early and seek the appropriate treatment. Below, I've highlighted some key signs to keep in mind.

- **Severe pain**: If you experience severe and persistent pain in your legs, especially where varicose veins are located, this may be a sign of varicose-related complications, such as deep vein thrombosis (DVT). DVT occurs when a blood clot forms in the deep veins of the legs, which can block blood flow and cause severe pain and tenderness.

- **Swelling**: Swelling in the legs and ankles can be a sign of fluid accumulation, known as edema. In cases of varicose veins, swelling may indicate venous insufficiency, which occurs when the veins cannot efficiently pump blood back to the heart. Venous insufficiency can cause a buildup of fluid in the surrounding tissues, resulting in swelling.

- **Skin changes**: Varicose veins can affect the health of the skin on your legs. If you notice changes in the skin, such as redness, peeling, itching, or the appearance of ulcers, this may indicate complications related to varicose veins. The skin around varicose veins may also become thicker and harder due to blood pooling and inadequate blood flow.

- **Bleeding**: If varicose veins rupture or become damaged, they can cause bleeding. Although bleeding from varicose veins is usually mild, it can be more significant and require immediate medical attention. If you experience persistent or heavy bleeding, it is crucial to seek immediate medical attention to control the situation and prevent further complications.

• **Venous ulcers**: Venous ulcers are open wounds or sores that form on the skin due to poor blood circulation in the legs. These ulcers are more common in people with advanced varicose veins and can be difficult to heal. Venous ulcers usually occur near the ankles and are painful. If you develop a venous ulcer, you should seek medical attention for proper treatment and infection prevention.

• **Muscle cramps**: Muscle cramps in the legs can be a sign of complications related to varicose veins. Poor blood circulation in the affected veins can cause a lack of nutrients and oxygen to the muscles, leading to painful cramps. If you experience recurring muscle cramps in your legs, especially at night, it may indicate underlying vein problems.

• **Feeling of heaviness or fatigue in the legs**: Varicose veins can cause a feeling of heaviness or fatigue in the legs, especially after prolonged periods of standing or sitting. This is due to the accumulation of blood in the dilated veins, which hinders venous return and causes a feeling of tiredness in the legs. If you experience this sensation persistently or if it worsens over time, it is advisable to seek medical attention.

• **Changes in the appearance of varicose veins**: If varicose veins suddenly change appearance, such as becoming more significant, more painful, or more prominent, it may be a sign of complications. These changes may indicate increased pressure in the veins or the formation of a blood clot inside them. Pay attention to changes in varicose veins and consult a physician if you notice any changes.

• **Tenderness or pain when touching varicose veins**: If varicose veins become tender or painful when touched, this may be a sign of inflammation or irritation in the veins. Excessive pressure or trauma to the varicose veins can trigger these symptoms and, in some cases, may indicate the presence of a complication such as thrombophlebitis, which is inflammation of a vein due to clot formation.

• **Changes in skin temperature**: Varicose veins can affect the skin temperature on the legs. If you notice that the skin around varicose veins feels warmer or cooler than the rest, this may indicate a circulatory problem. Changes in temperature could be a sign of blocked or altered blood flow in the affected veins.

• **Changes in skin coloration**: In advanced cases of varicose veins, the accumulation of blood in the veins can lead to changes in skin coloration. You may notice brown spots or areas of dark pigmentation around the varicose veins. These changes in coloration may indicate poor blood circulation and could be a sign of chronic venous insufficiency.

• **Itching or burning sensation**: Varicose veins may cause an itching or burning sensation in the skin of the legs. This may be due to blood pooling, swelling, or irritation in the affected veins. Itching can be especially intense after standing for a long time or in hot climates.

• **Bleeding or hemorrhage**: If varicose veins are injured or ruptured, they can cause bleeding or hemorrhage. If you experience persistent or heavy bleeding from varicose veins, you should seek medical attention immediately. Excessive bleeding could be a sign of a serious complication and may require urgent medical treatment.

• **Appearance of varicose veins in new areas**: If you notice the appearance of new varicose veins in areas other than the legs, such as the abdomen or pelvic area, this may be a sign of more serious problems in the venous system. These varicose veins may be related to chronic venous insufficiency or other underlying medical conditions and require proper medical evaluation.

• **Difficulty walking or moving**: In advanced cases of varicose veins, poor blood circulation and fluid accumulation in the legs can make movement difficult and cause weakness or pain when walking. If you experience difficulty walking or moving due to varicose veins, it is important to seek medical attention to receive proper treatment and prevent further complications.

It's important to keep in mind that warning signs can vary from person to person and don't always indicate a serious condition. However, staying vigilant about any changes in your varicose veins is crucial for maintaining your health. If you notice any of these symptoms, don't hesitate to seek medical advice to address your doubts or concerns.

Timely diagnosis and treatment can make a world of difference. Not only does it help prevent complications, but it also significantly enhances your quality of life, empowering you to feel your best and enjoy each day with peace of mind. Your health and well-being should always come first!

FREQUENTLY ASKED QUESTIONS

Navigating the intricate world of health can feel overwhelming, especially when faced with a diagnosis that affects both physical and emotional well-being. In such moments, many questions naturally arise: What does this mean for me? What options are available? How will my daily life change? Uncertainty and concern are common. Here, you'll discover practical and direct insights to help you make confident, informed choices.

This chapter was created to offer support and provide clear, straightforward tools to guide you through this journey. In today's era of abundant information, distinguishing reliable knowledge from content that might cause confusion is vital. With this in mind, I've compiled evidence-based guidance to help you navigate uncertainty with greater clarity.

The format of this resource prioritizes accessibility, addressing common concerns faced by individuals and families alike. Each explanation is concise, clear, and aimed at empowering you to make decisions that align with your overall well-being.

While the material here is designed to assist, it is not a substitute for personalized advice from healthcare professionals. Consulting your doctor for guidance tailored to your specific needs remains essential, especially to address challenges unique to your situation.

Through these pages, my goal is to foster calm, confidence, and reassurance so that you can approach your circumstances with strength and resolve. I hope this resource inspires you and provides the valuable tools necessary to manage your health effectively and confidently.

112 FAQs About Varicose Veins

1. What are varicose veins?

Varicose veins are dilated, twisted veins that develop when the valves in the veins do not function properly, causing blood to pool.

2. What are the common symptoms of varicose veins?

Symptoms include visible purple or blue veins, pain or heaviness in the legs, swelling, cramping, itching around the affected vein, and, in some cases, skin ulcers.

3. What factors increase the risk of developing varicose veins?

Risk factors include family history, advanced age, being female, pregnancy, obesity, standing or sitting for long periods, and lack of exercise.

4. How are varicose veins diagnosed?

Physical examination is used to diagnose; a Doppler ultrasound is often used to evaluate blood flow and vein structure.

5. What medical treatments are available?

Treatments include lifestyle changes, compression stockings, sclerotherapy, laser therapy, radiofrequency ablation, and, in severe cases, surgery.

6. When should you see your doctor for varicose veins?

A doctor should be consulted if you experience persistent pain, swelling, skin changes, or varicose veins that affect your quality of life.

7. Do varicose veins disappear on their own?

Varicose veins do not usually disappear without treatment, although some symptoms often improve with lifestyle changes and conservative treatments.

8. What are spider veins, and how do they differ from varicose veins?

Spider veins are small dilated veins that appear near the skin's surface, usually red, blue, or purple. Unlike varicose veins, they are generally painless and smaller.

9. Is it safe to fly in an airplane if I have varicose veins?
Yes, flying is safe, but certain precautions, such as wearing compression stockings, moving periodically during the flight, and staying hydrated, are recommended to reduce the risk of complications such as deep vein thrombosis.

10. How do hormones affect varicose veins?
Hormones, especially estrogen and progesterone, can weaken vein walls and affect valve function, which can increase the likelihood of developing varicose veins, especially during pregnancy or with the use of hormonal contraceptives.

11. Do oral contraceptives affect the development of varicose veins?
Some oral contraceptives may increase the risk of developing varicose veins due to hormonal changes that affect the vein wall and blood clotting.

12. Can men also have varicose veins?
Yes, although varicose veins are more common in women, men can also develop them due to genetic factors, lifestyle, or underlying medical conditions.

13. Can varicose veins be prevented?
Although not always preventable, maintaining a healthy weight, including a balanced diet, exercising regularly, avoiding smoking, elevating the legs, and avoiding long periods of standing or sitting, reduces the risk of developing varicose veins.

14. How can varicose veins be prevented in office work?
Maintaining proper sitting posture, such as avoiding crossing your legs, keeping your feet flat on the floor, getting up and moving regularly, stretching your legs, using a footrest, and wearing compression stockings if necessary, can improve circulation and reduce pressure in the veins, helping to prevent the development of varicose veins.

15. How does a sedentary lifestyle affect venous health?
A sedentary lifestyle can decrease blood flow in the legs, increase venous pressure, and increase the risk of developing

varicose veins. Regular movement is crucial to maintaining good circulation.

16. What role does regular exercise play?

Regular exercise, such as walking, swimming, or cycling, strengthens leg muscles, improves circulation, and often reduces the symptoms of varicose veins or helps prevent them. However, high-impact exercise or excessive lifting should be avoided if it causes discomfort.

17. Is it possible to do intensive exercise?

Yes, it is possible, but it is important to choose activities that do not put excessive pressure on the legs, such as swimming or cycling, and to wear compression stockings during exercise if necessary.

18. How can aquatic exercise benefit?

Aquatic exercise, such as swimming or water aerobics, provides a low-impact environment that strengthens muscles, improves circulation, reduces swelling, and relieves pressure on veins, benefiting people with varicose veins.

19. How can cycling help prevent or relieve varicose veins?

Cycling is an exercise that activates the leg muscles and strengthens the calves, improving blood circulation and reducing pressure on the veins, which can prevent the development of varicose veins and relieve their symptoms.

20. How can walking help prevent and manage varicose veins?

Walking is an excellent exercise that improves leg circulation, strengthens the calf muscles, and helps prevent blood pooling in the veins.

21. How can stretching exercises benefit?

Stretching exercises improve flexibility and blood flow, reduce venous pressure, and relieve leg tension, which is beneficial for people with varicose veins.

22. How can physical therapy help?

Physical therapy can include specific exercises to improve circulation, massage to reduce swelling, techniques to strengthen leg muscles, and education on leg care, all of which contribute to managing and preventing varicose veins.

23. How can diet influence venous health and varicose veins?

A diet rich in fiber, vitamins, flavonoids, and antioxidants and low in salt improves vascular health, helps maintain a healthy weight, improves circulation, and reduces swelling. This contributes to better venous health and helps prevent the development or worsening of varicose veins.

24. Does wearing high heels affect varicose veins?

Wearing high heels for prolonged periods can hinder venous circulation and contribute to developing or worsening varicose veins. By altering the normal functioning of the calf muscles, high heels can also make venous return more difficult.

25. How can appropriate shoes prevent the worsening of varicose veins?

Wearing comfortable and supportive shoes, especially those with good arch support, can reduce pressure on the legs and improve circulation, helping to prevent the worsening of varicose veins.

26. Can prolonged use of tight pantyhose cause varicose veins?

Tight pantyhoses not explicitly designed for therapeutic compression do not cause varicose veins but can hinder circulation if they are too tight.

27. Can varicose veins be treated with natural remedies?

Natural remedies, such as applying cold compresses, consuming plant extracts such as horse chestnut, and elevating the legs, help alleviate the symptoms. The corresponding chapter will discuss these remedies in detail.

28. Can varicose veins develop in other parts of the body?

Although most common in the legs, varicose veins can occur in other areas, such as the esophagus, rectum (hemorrhoids), and scrotum (varicocele).

29. What are the symptoms of esophageal varices?
Esophageal varices are dilated veins in the esophagus that can cause bleeding. Symptoms may include vomiting blood, black stools, and dizziness. They are not related to varicose veins in the legs but are a severe medical condition that requires immediate attention.

30. How do varicose veins affect quality of life?
Varicose veins can cause physical discomfort, such as pain, swelling, itching, and leg fatigue. In some cases, they can limit mobility and affect the overall quality of life. Due to their visible appearance, varicose veins can also affect self-esteem and confidence.

31. Can varicose veins cause a burning sensation in the legs?
Yes, varicose veins can cause a burning sensation in the legs due to the accumulation of blood and pressure in the affected veins.

32. Can varicose veins cause changes in skin color?
Yes, varicose veins can cause changes in skin color, such as brown or reddish spots, due to venous hypertension and damage to the surrounding tissues.

33. What is venous hypertension, and how is it related to varicose veins?
Venous hypertension is increased pressure in the veins caused by defective venous valves. This additional pressure can lead to the development of varicose veins and other venous problems.

34. What is venous dermatitis or venous stasis dermatitis?
Venous dermatitis is an inflammation of the skin caused by poor venous circulation. It can occur in people with varicose veins and is characterized by itching, redness, and peeling of the skin due to the accumulation of blood and fluid.

35. What is hyperpigmentation of the skin related to varicose veins?

It is the darkening of the skin, usually on the lower legs, caused by the accumulation of blood and the deposit of hemoglobin breakdown products due to venous insufficiency.

36. Are varicose veins dangerous?

Although generally not dangerous, varicose veins can cause complications such as ulcers, superficial thrombophlebitis, or bleeding if not adequately treated.

37. What are the risks of not treating varicose veins long-term?

If left untreated, varicose veins can lead to severe complications such as venous ulcers, deep vein thrombosis, infections, and permanent skin changes.

38. What are venous ulcers, and how are they related to varicose veins?

Venous ulcers are open sores that develop on the skin, usually on the lower legs, due to poor venous circulation. They are common in people with varicose veins or chronic venous insufficiency. Without proper treatment, venous ulcers are usually painful and difficult to heal.

39. What is deep vein thrombosis, and how is it related to varicose veins?

Deep vein thrombosis (DVT) is the formation of a blood clot in a deep vein, usually in the legs. Although superficial varicose veins do not cause DVT, chronic venous insufficiency may increase the risk.

40. What is a post-thrombotic syndrome, and how is it related to varicose veins?

Post-thrombotic syndrome is a complication that can occur after deep vein thrombosis (DVT). It is characterized by pain, swelling, and varicose veins, which result from damage to the venous valves and obstruction of blood flow.

41. What is phlebitis, and how is it different from varicose veins?

Phlebitis is the inflammation of a vein, which can be superficial or deep. It can occur in varicose veins and cause pain, redness, and tenderness in the affected area. It is often associated with blood clots, while varicose veins are dilated and tortuous due to valvular insufficiency.

42. What is superficial thrombophlebitis, and how is it related to varicose veins?
Superficial thrombophlebitis is the inflammation of a vein near the skin's surface due to a blood clot. Unlike varicose veins, which are dilated veins, thrombophlebitis is usually painful.

43. What is chronic venous insufficiency, and how is it related to varicose veins?
Chronic venous insufficiency is when the veins have difficulty returning blood to the heart. This results in swelling, pain, skin changes, and varicose veins due to blood reflux and prolonged venous pressure.

44. What is deep venous insufficiency?
Deep venous insufficiency is a condition in which the valves in the deep veins of the legs do not function properly. This causes blood to pool, leading to more severe symptoms than superficial varicose veins.

45. Can varicose veins be hereditary?
The predisposition to develop varicose veins can be hereditary. If one or both parents have varicose veins, the risk of their children developing them is higher, although lifestyle also plays a part.

46. How does genetics influence the development of varicose veins?
Genetics can play an essential role in the predisposition to develop varicose veins. Due to hereditary weakness in the vein walls or valves, people with a family history are more likely to develop varicose veins.

47. Does pregnancy always cause varicose veins?
Not always, although it increases the risk.

48. Is it possible to prevent varicose veins during pregnancy?

Although not wholly preventable, wearing compression stockings, maintaining a healthy weight, elevating the legs, and exercising regularly can reduce the risk of developing varicose veins during pregnancy.

49. What is the impact of pregnancy on varicose veins?
Pregnancy increases the risk of varicose veins due to hormonal changes, increased blood volume, and pressure from the uterus on the pelvic veins, although they often improve after delivery.

50. How can varicose veins be prevented from worsening during pregnancy?
To prevent varicose veins from worsening during pregnancy, it is recommended to wear compression stockings, exercise moderately, elevate the legs, and avoid standing or sitting for long periods.

51. How can elevating the legs help with the symptoms?
Elevating the legs above the heart level several times a day can reduce pressure in the leg veins, improve venous return, and relieve swelling and discomfort associated with varicose veins.

52. How can using leg elevation pillows during rest help people with varicose veins?
Elevating the legs with pillows while resting helps improve blood flow back to the heart, reduce swelling, and relieve pressure on the veins affected by varicose veins.

53. What is pelvic congestion syndrome?
Pelvic congestion syndrome is a condition in which the veins in the pelvis become dilated and can cause chronic pain. It is related to pelvic varicose veins and may be more common in women who have had multiple pregnancies.

54. Is it possible for varicose veins to cause sleep problems?
The discomfort and night cramps associated with varicose veins can interfere with sleep, affecting rest and quality of life.

55. Can varicose veins cause nocturnal leg cramps?

Yes, varicose veins can contribute to night cramps due to poor circulation and blood pooling in the affected veins. Keeping the legs elevated and using compression can help alleviate these symptoms.

56. What is compression therapy, and how is it used to treat varicose veins?

Compression therapy involves using compression stockings or bandages to improve blood flow in the legs, reduce swelling, and relieve the symptoms of varicose veins. The stockings apply graduated pressure, being tighter at the ankle and tapering upward.

57. What are compression stockings, and how do they help with varicose veins?

Compression stockings are elastic garments that apply pressure to the legs to improve blood flow and reduce swelling, pain, and heaviness associated with varicose veins.

58. What is compression bandaging, and how is it used to manage varicose veins?

Compression bandaging involves wrapping the legs with elastic bandages to apply pressure, improve venous circulation, and reduce swelling and pain associated with varicose veins.

59. Can heat affect varicose veins?

Yes, heat can dilate the veins and worsen the symptoms of varicose veins, so it is advisable to avoid prolonged hot baths and protect yourself from extreme heat.

60. How does being overweight or obese affect varicose veins?

Being overweight puts additional pressure on the leg veins, hinders venous return, and weakens the venous valves, contributing to the development and worsening of varicose veins and venous insufficiency.

61. What role does hydration play in venous health?

Staying well hydrated helps improve blood circulation and can prevent swelling and heaviness in the legs, which benefits people with varicose veins.

62. What impact does smoking have on varicose veins?
Smoking damages blood vessels and affects circulation, contributing to the development and worsening of varicose veins.

63. Does alcohol consumption affect varicose veins?
Excessive alcohol consumption can dilate veins and worsen varicose vein symptoms, as well as contribute to dehydration and other circulatory problems, increasing the risk of complications.

64. How does aging influence the development of varicose veins?
With age, the veins tend to lose elasticity, and the valves may weaken, which increases the risk of developing varicose veins due to the accumulation of blood in them.

65. Is it advisable to massage legs with varicose veins?
Gentle massage can improve circulation and relieve discomfort in legs with varicose veins, but direct pressure on prominent or swollen veins should be avoided.

66. How can therapeutic massages help?
Therapeutic massage can improve circulation, reduce swelling, and relieve muscle tension in the legs, which may alleviate some symptoms associated with varicose veins. However, direct pressure on varicose veins must be avoided.

67. Can varicose veins affect fertility?
There is no direct evidence that varicose veins affect fertility, but related conditions, such as varicocele in men, may impact fertility. In women, pelvic varicose veins may be associated with chronic pelvic pain.

68. Can yoga practice help with varicose veins?
Yoga often improves circulation, strengthens leg muscles, reduces venous pressure, and increases flexibility, which can alleviate some symptoms of varicose veins. Postures that elevate the legs are often beneficial.

69. Can stress influence the development of varicose

veins?
Chronic stress can affect vascular health by increasing blood pressure and causing inflammation, which may influence the development and worsening of varicose veins. Stress management techniques like meditation and yoga can benefit venous health.

70. How can relaxation techniques help?
Relaxation techniques, such as meditation or deep breathing, help reduce stress and improve overall blood flow, positively affecting venous health.

71. How can deep breathing techniques help?
Deep breathing improves venous return to the heart by increasing pressure in the abdomen and chest, which can help relieve pressure in the leg veins.

72. How are varicose veins related to restless legs syndrome?
Due to blood pooling and high blood pressure, people with varicose veins may experience a restless feeling in their legs, similar to restless leg syndrome.

73. Is it possible to use makeup to hide varicose veins?
Makeup or concealer products can help conceal the appearance of varicose veins, although they do not treat the underlying cause.

74. How are varicose veins different from incompetent perforating veins?
Incompetent perforating veins connect the superficial venous system to the deep venous system and, when unqualified, can contribute to the development of varicose veins by allowing blood to reflux.

75. How do the hormonal changes of menopause influence varicose veins?
During menopause, decreased estrogen levels can affect the elasticity of the veins, increasing the risk of developing or worsening varicose veins.

76. What role do antioxidants play in vein health?
Antioxidants in foods such as fruits and vegetables help protect vein walls from oxidative damage, strengthen veins, and reduce the risk of developing varicose veins.

77. How can cold showers help with varicose veins?
Cold showers can help constrict blood vessels and improve circulation, temporarily relieving the swelling and discomfort associated with varicose veins.

78. What is hydrotherapy, and how can it help varicose veins?
Hydrotherapy involves using water at different temperatures to improve circulation and reduce swelling. Contrast baths (alternating hot and cold water) can be particularly helpful in improving circulation in the legs, helping to relieve the symptoms of varicose veins.

79. What role does collagen play in venous health and the prevention of varicose veins?
Collagen is an essential protein for the structural integrity of blood vessels. Maintaining adequate levels of collagen can help strengthen vein walls and prevent the dilation that leads to varicose veins.

80. What is the role of vitamin C in venous health?
Vitamin C is essential for producing collagen, strengthening vein walls, and improving circulation, which may help prevent or reduce varicose veins.

81. How can the use of supplements help venous health?
Some supplements, such as those containing horse chestnut extracts or flavonoids, help improve circulation and strengthen vein walls, which can help manage varicose veins. We will see this in the chapter "Nutritional Supplements".

82. What is May-Thurner syndrome, and its relation to varicose veins?
May-Thurner syndrome occurs when the right iliac artery compresses the left iliac vein. This can cause swelling, pain, and the development of varicose veins in the left leg.

83. How can intermittent pneumatic compression help?
When used regularly, this treatment involves inflating and deflating a device around the legs to improve blood circulation, reduce swelling, and relieve symptoms of varicose veins.

84. How can using essential oils benefit?
Some essential oils, such as cypress or rosemary, help improve circulation and reduce swelling when applied topically with gentle massage. However, diluting essential oils and performing a sensitivity test before using them extensively is always important.

85. What is cupping therapy, and can it be helpful for varicose veins?
Cupping therapy is an alternative medicine technique that uses cups to create skin suction, helping improve blood circulation.

86. What is Klippel-Trenaunay syndrome, and its relation to varicose veins?
Klippel-Trenaunay syndrome is a rare congenital condition characterized by vascular malformations, varicose veins, and soft tissue and bone overgrowth, which can cause significant venous complications.

87. What is dermatoliposclerosis, and how is it related to varicose veins?
Dermatoliposclerosis is a condition that develops due to chronic venous insufficiency. It causes the skin and underlying tissues to become hardened and discolored. Untreated varicose veins can contribute to this condition.

88. What is the CHIVA technique for treating varicose veins?
The CHIVA (Conservative and Hemodynamic Cure of Ambulatory Venous Insufficiency) technique is a conservative approach that seeks to preserve venous function by correcting blood flow without eliminating veins.

89. Which health professionals treat varicose veins?
Varicose veins can be treated by phlebologists, vascular surgeons, and dermatologists specializing in vascular treatments.

90. What is phlebography, and how is it used to diagnose varicose veins?
Phlebography is a diagnostic imaging procedure in which a contrast medium is injected into the veins to visualize their structure and function on an X-ray. It is used to evaluate complex cases of varicose veins and venous insufficiency.

91. Is surgery to treat varicose veins painful?
Most modern procedures to treat varicose veins are minimally invasive and are performed under local anesthesia, which minimizes pain and recovery time.

92. Is it necessary to fast before varicose vein procedures?
Depending on the type of procedure, the physician may recommend fasting beforehand, especially if any kind of anesthesia is administered.

93. What is the recovery time after a procedure to treat varicose veins?
Recovery time varies depending on the type of procedure, but most modern treatments allow a quick return to normal activities.

94. What postoperative care is necessary after treating varicose veins?
Care depends on the procedure. In some interventions, it is recommended to wear compression stockings, avoid prolonged exposure to the sun, and hydrate adequately. Follow medical indications to ensure optimal recovery.

95. What is transillumination, and how is it used to treat varicose veins?
Transillumination is a technique that uses a special light to visualize varicose veins under the skin. It helps to guide treatment procedures such as sclerotherapy or phyto-extraction.

96. What is ambulatory phlebectomy, and how is it performed?
Ambulatory phlebectomy is a minor surgical procedure in which varicose veins are removed through small incisions in

the skin. It is performed under local anesthesia, is effective in treating superficial veins, and allows people to go home the same day.

97. What is phytoextraction, and when is it used?

Phleboextraction is a surgical procedure involving removing a varicose vein through small incisions. It is generally used to treat large and severe varicose veins.

98. What is venous stripping, and how is it used to treat varicose veins?

Venous stripping is a surgical procedure in which a long varicose vein is removed using a particular device. This treatment is performed under anesthesia and is used to remove severely affected veins.

99. What is ultrasound-guided sclerosis or sclerotherapy?

It is a technique in which ultrasound is used to visualize varicose veins during sclerotherapy, allowing the physician to accurately inject the sclerosing solution into veins that are not visible to the naked eye, improving the accuracy and effectiveness of the treatment.

100. How are sclerotherapy procedures performed?

Sclerotherapy involves injecting a solution into the affected vein. This causes the vein walls to adhere and eventually close, redirecting blood flow to healthy veins.

101. What is sclerotherapy or foam sclerosis therapy?

Foam sclerotherapy is a procedure in which a foam solution is injected into varicose veins to close them and redirect blood flow to healthy veins.

102. What is chemical sclerosis, and how is it different from foam sclerosis?

Chemical sclerosis uses a liquid solution to treat varicose veins, while foam sclerosis uses a foam version of the sclerosing agent.

103. What is microsclerosis therapy, or microsclero-therapy, and what is it used for?

Microsclerotherapy is a technique for treating spider veins and small varicose veins. It involves injecting a sclerosing solution with fine needles to close the affected veins.

104. What is endovenous laser sclerosis, and how is it used to treat varicose veins?

EVLT is a minimally invasive procedure that uses laser energy to close varicose veins from the inside. It is performed under ultrasound guidance and effectively treats more prominent veins.

105. What is transdermal or transcutaneous laser therapy, and how is it used to treat varicose veins?

Transdermal laser therapy involves externally applying a laser to the skin to treat small superficial varicose veins, such as spider veins. The laser heats and destroys the veins without the need for incisions or injections. This non-invasive procedure can improve the appearance of the skin.

106. What is laser photocoagulation, and how is it used to treat spider veins?

Laser photocoagulation is a procedure that uses laser energy to heat and close spider veins. It is a non-invasive treatment that can improve the appearance of the skin.

107. What is microwave treatment, and how is it used to treat varicose veins?

Microwave treatment uses microwave energy to heat and close varicose veins. It is a relatively new and minimally invasive technique that offers another option for treating varicose veins.

108. What is infrared therapy, and how is it used to treat varicose veins?

Infrared therapy uses infrared light to penetrate the skin, improve circulation, relieve pain, and reduce swelling. Although promising, its effectiveness, specifically for varicose veins, requires further research.

109. What is glue injection therapy, and how is it used to treat varicose veins?

Glue injection therapy involves using a medical adhesive to

close varicose veins. It is a quick and effective procedure that does not require heat or incisions.

110. What is ozone therapy, and how is it applied to varicose veins?

Ozone therapy involves injecting a mixture of oxygen and ozone into the affected veins to improve circulation and reduce inflammation. However, its effectiveness for varicose veins is not well-documented scientifically.

111. What is angiogenesis, and how does it relate to varicose veins?

Angiogenesis is the process of new blood vessel formation. In the context of varicose veins, angiogenesis may contribute to the formation of new abnormal veins after specific treatments.

112. Can varicose veins recur after treatment?

Yes, varicose veins can recur after any treatment, mainly if the underlying causes or risk factors are not addressed. Medical follow-up and maintaining a healthy lifestyle are essential.

SUGGESTED PRACTICAL PLAN

Here's a practical and detailed plan with effective steps to help you treat varicose veins. This comprehensive approach is designed to guide you, step by step, toward restoring your well-being. Let's get started!

• **Understand the Origin**: Identifying the causes of your varicose veins is the first and most critical step. Understanding the factors behind their development will empower you to take proactive measures to prevent and minimize these issues. For more detailed insights, refer to the chapter "Varicose Veins", specifically the sections "Causes" and "Symptom Relief and Prevention". These sections will prove to be incredibly valuable!

• **Strengthen Your Body with Supplements**: Adding nutritional supplements into your daily routine can play a pivotal role in your recovery. Supplements help enhance the health of your veins from within, accelerating the healing process. In the next chapter, you'll find an in-depth guide to the most effective supplements, along with safe usage tips to achieve the best possible results.

• **Harness the Power of Medicinal Plants**: Nature offers powerful solutions for vein health. Medicinal plants and phytotherapy treatments can be excellent allies, helping to alleviate discomfort and improve vein function. Explore the chapter "Medicinal Plants" to discover targeted solutions that can support your recovery journey.

• **Embrace a Proper Diet**: The food you eat daily has a direct and meaningful impact on the health of your veins. A well-balanced diet can become your strongest ally in fighting varicose veins, while certain foods may slow down your progress. That's why paying attention to your diet is essential. Refer to the chapters "Foods That Transform" and "Juices and Smoothies" to access a list of beneficial foods and over 50 delicious, nutrient-packed recipes designed to nurture your venous system. Additionally, you'll find a dedicated guide to special juices that will help fortify your veins and enhance your overall well-being. Remember, your health starts with what's on your plate!

• **Review the Impact of Medications**: If you suspect that any medication may be worsening your symptoms, it's crucial to bring this up with your doctor. This is particularly relevant in the case of hormonal contraceptives or any treatment that could affect blood circulation. Your healthcare provider can help assess the situation and determine if there are better alternatives tailored to your needs.

• **Lifestyle Adjustments**: Making small yet meaningful changes to your daily routine can go a long way in managing and improving your varicose veins. Refer to the practical strategies detailed in the "Varicose Veins" chapter, especially in the sections "Symptom Relief and Prevention" and "Additional Tips". Whether it's adopting simple habits or implementing more significant lifestyle shifts, every step you take contributes to improving your overall health.

• **Add Movement to Your Daily Routine**: Engaging in regular physical activity is key to boosting blood circulation and enhancing vein health. Activities such as walking, swimming, cycling, or dancing are not only great for your legs but also improve your overall well-being. Incorporating movement into your day-to-day life can lead to noticeable benefits for your health—and the best part is, it's something you can truly enjoy!

Additional Resources
If you're experiencing varicose veins alongside other conditions such as hemorrhoids or constipation, you may find valuable remedies and advice in my books:

- **HEMORRHOIDS**. Foods, Supplements, and Medicinal Plants
- **CONSTIPATION**. Foods, Supplements, and Medicinal Plants

Remember: Every Step Counts

Every small change you make contributes to better vein health. While the results may not always be immediate, the consistent effort you put in will lead to noticeable improvements over time. Never underestimate the positive impact of your daily choices, as you hold the power to transform your overall well-being.

Believe in yourself, and take the first step toward healthier veins today!

NUTRITIONAL SUPPLEMENTS

"Your true wealth is health"
(Ralph Waldo Emerson)

Nutritional supplements have become a valuable ally in the pursuit of better health and an enhanced quality of life. These options–available in various user-friendly formats such as tablets, capsules, powders, or easily consumable liquids–are purposefully designed to complement your daily nutrition by delivering essential nutrients that can be challenging to obtain through regular meals alone. Packed with powerful components like vitamins, minerals, amino acids, antioxidants, and other bioactive compounds, these supplements are expertly formulated in precise proportions to meet the unique needs of every individual–even when the demands are high. Whether you're navigating restrictive diets, facing nutritional gaps, or coping with increased physical or mental demands, supplements can provide the extra support your body needs.

Beyond simply filling in nutritional gaps, supplements offer an array of tailored benefits to suit diverse lifestyles and health challenges. They can help boost energy, improve physical performance, support those managing fast-paced lives, and provide practical solutions for staying balanced and resilient. Their significance often becomes even more apparent during times of illness, specific health conditions, or chronic issues. In these situations, supplements do more than complement a diet–they can actively help restore altered functions, ease symptoms, and assist in more complex recovery processes. They serve as companions in the pursuit of health, helping you sustain and rebuild your vitality.

Effectively integrating supplements into your routine requires thoughtful use grounded in science and, when needed, professional guidance. By understanding their benefits and approaching them with care, supplements can evolve into powerful tools for improving your overall well-being in a sustainable and meaningful way. Remember–every step you take toward caring for your body is a step closer to feeling stronger, more energized, and more capable of facing life's challenges with confidence. Take that step today. Your path to better health begins with small but impactful choices!

Essential Precautions

Understanding the risks associated with supplements is vital, as they can sometimes cause side effects, have contraindications, or interact with medications. It's important to thoroughly review the potential adverse effects detailed at the end of this chapter. Take a moment to assess your overall health and avoid any supplements that could conflict with the medications you're currently taking or exacerbate existing medical conditions. Prioritizing this step ensures a safer and more effective approach to improving your well-being.

Nutritional Supplements and Varicose Veins

In today's fast-paced world, we are constantly challenged to balance our responsibilities while prioritizing our well-being. Too often, the hectic nature of daily life leads us to overlook essential aspects of our health. Among these, varicose veins have become a prevalent issue, affecting a significant portion of the population. These swollen and twisted veins, most commonly found in the legs, not only influence our appearance but also cause physical discomfort, which can significantly impact our quality of life.

Understanding the most effective ways to take care of your veins can make a profound difference, and this is where nutritional supplements play a vital role. This chapter is dedicated to exploring how a diet enriched with specific supplements can serve as a powerful ally in managing varicose veins.

An increasing body of research highlights the benefits of proper supplementation in strengthening blood vessel walls, improving circulation, and reducing the discomfort associated with this condition.

In the following pages, you will discover the most highly recommended supplements, their modes of action, and the potential advantages they offer. Clear and practical dosage guidelines are also provided, helping you seamlessly incorporate these supplements into your daily routine. To make your exploration easier, the supplements are presented in alphabetical order.

By making small yet meaningful changes to your nutritional habits, you can support your body, alleviate discomfort, and improve the health of your veins. Let's begin this journey to better care for your well-being!

Diosmin

Diosmin is a flavonoid commonly used for the treatment of varicose veins and other issues related to venous circulation. Its main benefits include:

• Improves Circulation: Diosmin helps strengthen blood vessel walls and improve blood flow. This can relieve symptoms associated with varicose veins, such as heaviness, pain, and swelling in the legs.

• Reduces Inflammation: Diosmin has anti-inflammatory properties that help reduce swelling in veins affected by varicose veins. This alleviates discomfort and improves the appearance of the legs.

• Strengthens Veins: Diosmin promotes the synthesis of collagen and elastin, two key components of vein walls. This strengthens the veins and makes them more resistant, thus decreasing the likelihood of new varicose veins forming.

Dosage:
The standard dose ranges from 500 mg to 1000 mg per day.

Posology:
It is recommended that diosmin be taken in two or three

doses, preferably with food, to improve absorption and reduce possible gastrointestinal effects.

Onset of Action:
Effects are generally observed within 1 to 2 weeks of continuous treatment.

Maximum Time of Continuous Use:
While the maximum time of continuous use is not strictly defined, many studies suggest that it can be used continuously for 3 to 6 months. Consult a health professional if you use it for more than 6 consecutive months.

Escin

Escin is a natural compound found in the seeds of the horse chestnut (Aesculus hippocastanum) and is widely used in the treatment of varicose veins and other venous disorders. Some of its benefits include:

• Improved Circulation: Escin helps strengthen blood vessel walls and reduce capillary permeability. This improves venous circulation, reduces congestion, and relieves symptoms such as swelling, heaviness, and pain.

• Anti-inflammatory Action: Escin has anti-inflammatory properties that reduce inflammation in the veins. This alleviates discomfort and improves the appearance of the legs.

• Protection of the Venous System: Escin strengthens veins and capillaries, helping prevent the formation of new varicose veins and reducing the risk of complications, such as venous ulcers.

Dosage:
The typical dose ranges from 150 to 300 mg of pure escin daily.

Posology:
Escin should be taken twice with meals to improve

absorption and minimize possible gastrointestinal effects.

Onset of Action:
Effects are generally observed within 1 to 2 weeks of continuous treatment.

Maximum Time of Continuous Use:
Continued use is considered safe in the short to medium term (up to 6 months), but it is essential to follow a specialist's recommendations to determine the appropriate duration according to your individual needs.

Ginkgo biloba

Ginkgo biloba is a medicinal plant that has been used for hundreds of years in traditional Chinese medicine for its various therapeutic properties. While it has been primarily studied for its benefits on cerebral circulation and memory, its potential use in the treatment of varicose veins has also been explored. Below are some of the benefits of Ginkgo biloba for varicose veins:

• Improves circulation: Ginkgo biloba has vasodilating and antioxidant properties that enhance blood flow and micro-circulation. This helps alleviate the symptoms of varicose veins, such as heaviness and swelling in the legs.

• Strengthens blood vessels: Ginkgo biloba strengthens the walls of blood vessels, including veins, by promoting the production of collagen and elastin. This helps reduce vein fragility and prevents the formation of new varicose veins.

• Anti-inflammatory properties: Many studies indicate that Ginkgo biloba possesses anti-inflammatory properties, which help reduce inflammation in veins affected by varicose veins. This reduces discomfort and improves the appearance of the legs.

Dosage:
A dose of 120 to 240 mg of standardized extract per day is recommended.

Posology:
It is recommended to take it in 2 or 3 doses per day, preferably with meals, to improve gastrointestinal tolerance.

Onset of Action:
Effects are usually observed within 4 to 6 weeks of continuous use.

Maximum Time of Continuous Use:
Many studies conclude that it can be taken continuously for 6 months to 1 year. However, consulting with a healthcare professional to determine the appropriate duration according to your individual needs is advisable.

Hesperidin

Hesperidin is a flavonoid found in various citrus fruits, such as oranges and lemons. It has been studied for its benefits in the treatment of varicose veins and other venous disorders. Some of the benefits:

• Strengthens Blood Vessels: Hesperidin strengthens the walls of blood vessels, including veins, by increasing collagen production and improving the elasticity of vein walls. This helps reduce vein fragility and prevents the formation of new varicose veins.

• Improves Circulation: Hesperidin helps improve blood circulation and reduce venous congestion. Promoting better blood flow alleviates symptoms associated with varicose veins, such as heaviness and swelling.

• Antioxidant and Anti-Inflammatory Action: Hesperidin has antioxidant and anti-inflammatory properties that help reduce oxidative stress and inflammation in veins affected by varicose veins. This helps relieve discomfort and improve the appearance of the legs.

Dosage:
The usual dose ranges from 500 mg to 1000 mg per day.

Posology:
Hesperidin can be taken once or twice a day, with meals to improve absorption and reduce possible gastrointestinal effects.

Onset of Action:
Effects are typically observed within 2 to 4 weeks of continuous use.

Maximum Time of Continuous Use:
The maximum duration of continuous use is not established, but many experts suggest using it for up to 6 months. It is advisable to consult with a healthcare professional to determine the appropriate length of treatment based on your individual needs.

Horse Chestnut

It is a natural supplement widely used to relieve the symptoms of varicose veins. Its benefits are mainly due to its content of a compound called escin, which has anti-inflammatory and blood vessel-strengthening properties. Some of the benefits of varicose veins are mentioned below:

• Improves Circulation: It helps strengthen vein walls and reduces swelling, thereby improving circulation in legs affected by varicose veins.

• Relieves Pain and Heaviness: Its anti-inflammatory properties help reduce pain, swelling, and the feeling of heaviness associated with varicose veins.

• Strengthens Blood Vessels: The escin present in horse chestnut helps strengthen blood vessels and improve their elasticity, which can prevent the formation of new varicose veins and reduce the appearance of existing ones.

• Antioxidant: It contains antioxidants that protect tissues against free radical damage, which is beneficial for overall vascular health.

Dosage:
The typical daily dosage is 300 to 600 mg of standardized extract (containing 20% to 25% escin), which can be divided into smaller doses throughout the day.

Posology:
It is usually recommended to be taken in two or three divided doses throughout the day. Taking it with meals is advised to improve gastrointestinal tolerance and absorption.

Onset of Action:
Its effects are generally observed within 1 to 2 weeks of continuous use.

Maximum Time of Continuous Use:
Continued use should last 3 to 4 months. After this time, taking a break or consulting your physician to reevaluate the need for continued treatment is advisable.

Niacin or Vitamin B3

Niacin, also known as vitamin B3, is essential for the proper functioning of the body. It plays a vital role in the overall health of blood vessels and has some positive effects on varicose veins, such as:

• Improves blood circulation: niacin helps improve circulation by dilating blood vessels, which in turn can relieve pressure in the veins and improve blood flow.

• Cholesterol reduction: It is commonly used to help control blood cholesterol levels. Maintaining healthy cholesterol levels can prevent damage to blood vessels and improve overall cardiovascular health. This benefits varicose veins, as high cholesterol can contribute to their development.

• Antioxidant support: It has antioxidant properties, which means it helps protect cells and tissues from damage caused by free radicals. This may be relevant in the case of varicose veins, as oxidative stress plays a role in their formation and worsening.

Dosage:
It usually ranges from 500 mg to 2000 mg per day.

Posology:
It is recommended to take 1 or 2 doses. It is best taken with meals to reduce the risk of gastrointestinal side effects and minimize skin redness (a common side effect).

Onset of Action:
Effects are generally seen within 2 to 4 weeks of continuous use.

Maximum Time of Continuous Use:
It is not strictly defined, but many professionals conclude that it can be used continuously for 6 to 12 months under medical supervision. Regular monitoring is essential to evaluate effectiveness and any side effects.

Rutin

Rutin, or vitamin P, is a flavonoid found in several plants, such as buckwheat, chamomile, and citrus fruits. It has been studied for its benefits for vascular health, including varicose veins. Here are some benefits:

• Strengthening of Blood Vessels: Rutin has antioxidant and anti-inflammatory properties that help strengthen blood vessels. This is beneficial in the case of varicose veins, as these form when the veins weaken and dilate.

• Improved Circulation: Rutin helps improve blood circulation by increasing the strength and elasticity of blood vessels. This reduces pressure in the veins and improves blood flow.

• Reduced Inflammation: Rutin has anti-inflammatory properties that help reduce inflammation associated with varicose veins, relieving swelling and pain.

Dosage:
It usually ranges from 500 mg to 1000 mg per day.

Posology:
It can be taken with food once or twice a day to improve absorption and minimize possible gastrointestinal effects.

Onset of Action:
Effects are usually observed within 2 to 4 weeks of continuous use.

Maximum Duration of Continuous Use:
It is not strictly defined, but many experts suggest use for up to 6 months. It is advisable to consult with a healthcare professional to determine the appropriate duration based on your individual needs.

Vitamin C

It is an essential nutrient for the proper functioning of the human body. It plays a vital role in the overall health of the blood vessels and has positive effects on varicose veins, such as:

• Strengthening of Blood Vessels: Vitamin C is necessary for the synthesis of collagen, a protein that is part of the structure of blood vessels. Maintaining adequate levels of Vitamin C promotes collagen production and strengthens blood vessels, which helps prevent the weakening and dilation of veins.

• Antioxidant Action: Vitamin C is a potent antioxidant that helps protect cells and tissues from free radical damage. Oxidative stress contributes to the deterioration of blood vessels and worsens varicose veins. Consuming enough Vitamin C reduces this oxidative stress, promoting healthy blood vessels.

• Promotes Healing: Vitamin C is essential for the production of collagen, which is necessary for healing and tissue repair. In the case of varicose veins, Vitamin C helps accelerate the recovery of damaged tissues and promotes healing.

Dosage:

The recommended dosage may vary depending on individual needs but is generally between 500 to 2000 mg per day.

Posology:
It is recommended to be taken preferably during the day, with or without food.

Onset of Action:
Although the time of onset of action may vary, effects usually appear after a few weeks of continuous use.

Maximum Duration of Continuous Use:
Continued use is generally safe at adequate doses. If use is planned for more than six months in a row, it is recommended to follow the manufacturer's instructions or consult a specialist, especially if adverse effects occur.

Vitamin E

Vitamin E is a fat-soluble nutrient with antioxidant properties that plays a vital role in blood vessel health and has positive effects on varicose veins. Here are some of them:

• Antioxidant Action: Vitamin E is known for its ability to neutralize free radicals and reduce oxidative stress in the body. This is beneficial for varicose veins, as oxidative stress damages blood vessels and contributes to their weakening. By consuming enough Vitamin E, you help protect and strengthen blood vessels.

• Improved Circulation: Vitamin E improves blood circulation by dilating blood vessels and reducing platelet aggregation. This helps reduce pressure in the veins and improve blood flow, which can be beneficial for varicose veins.

• Anti-Inflammatory Properties: Vitamin E also has anti-inflammatory properties that help reduce inflammation and discomfort associated with varicose veins. This relieves symptoms such as swelling and pain.

Dosage:
It ranges from 100 to 500 IU (international units) per day. Higher doses may be used under medical supervision in some cases.

Posology:
Since it is a fat-soluble vitamin, it is recommended that it be taken in one or two doses with meals containing fat to improve its absorption.

Onset of Action:
Generally, antioxidant effects usually begin to be noticed within 1 to 3 weeks of continuous use, although specific benefits may take longer to become evident.

Maximum Duration of Continuous Use:
Vitamin E is generally safe for long-term use. However, it is recommended to stay within doses of 400 IU per day on a continuous basis without medical supervision. Some experts suggest continued use for up to 1 year, but it is essential to consult a healthcare professional to determine the appropriate duration based on your individual needs.

Adverse Effects, Contraindications, and Interactions

Before adding the recommended supplements to your routine, it is crucial to understand the potential side effects, contraindications, and interactions that may affect your health. Take the time to thoroughly review this section to ensure their safe and responsible use.

Diosmin

• **Side Effects:** It is generally considered safe and well-tolerated. However, mild effects, such as stomach upset, nausea, or diarrhea, may occur in some cases.

• **Contraindications**: Not recommended for use in pregnant or lactating women, except under medical supervision.

• **Interactions**: No significant drug interactions have been reported.

Escin

• **Side effects**: This may cause gastrointestinal discomfort, allergic skin reactions, and, in rare cases, headache or dizziness.

• **Contraindications**: It is not recommended for people allergic to horse chestnuts, with kidney problems, or during pregnancy and lactation.

• **Interactions**: May interact with anticoagulant drugs or drugs that affect circulation, increasing the risk of bleeding. It is essential to consult your doctor before use.

Ginkgo Biloba

• **Side Effects**: Some people may experience mild side effects, such as stomach upset, headache, dizziness, or allergic skin reactions.

• **Contraindications**: Its use should be avoided in people with bleeding disorders.

• **Interactions**: May interact with anticoagulant drugs, antiplatelet agents, anticonvulsants, antidepressants, and drugs to treat diabetes.

Hesperidin

• **Side Effects**: It is generally considered safe and well-tolerated. However, mild side effects, such as stomach upset or diarrhea, may occur in some cases.

• **Contraindications**: Not recommended for use in pregnant or lactating women, except under medical supervision.

• **Interactions**: No significant drug interactions have been reported.

Horse Chestnut

- **Side Effects**: Some people may experience stomach upset, nausea, dizziness, headache, or itchy skin due to horse chestnut consumption.

- **Contraindications**: Not recommended for use in pregnant or lactating women.

- **Interactions**: This may increase the risk of bleeding if combined with anticoagulants or antiplatelet drugs. It may also interact with medications used to treat diabetes and hypertension.

Niacin

- **Side Effects**: Common adverse effects of niacin include skin flushing, itching, a warm sensation, and facial flushing. It can also cause stomach problems such as nausea, vomiting, and diarrhea. In high doses, niacin can cause liver damage, blood sugar problems, and blood pressure issues.

- **Contraindications**: Not recommended for use in people with liver disease, gastric or intestinal ulcers, gout, or uncontrolled diabetes.

- **Interactions**: May interact with cholesterol medications, diabetes medications, blood pressure medications, and anticoagulant medications.

Rutin

- **Side Effects**: It is generally well-tolerated but may cause stomach upset, nausea, diarrhea, or headaches in some cases.

- **Contraindications**: Not recommended for use in pregnant or lactating women, except under medical supervision.

- **Interactions**: No significant drug interactions have been reported.

Vitamin C

- **Side Effects**: In high doses, it may cause stomach upset, diarrhea, nausea, or abdominal cramps. Some people may also experience heartburn or intestinal irritation.

• **Contraindications**: It is not recommended for people with renal disorders or chronic kidney disease. In addition, caution should be exercised in people with a history of kidney stones or glucose-6-phosphate dehydrogenase deficiency.

• **Interactions**: May interact with certain medications, such as anticoagulants, aspirin, cancer drugs, oral contraceptives, statins, and antipsychotics.

Vitamin E

• **Side Effects**: In high doses, it may cause stomach upset, diarrhea, headache, and fatigue.

• **Contraindications**: Not recommended for use in people with coagulation disorders or those taking anticoagulant drugs.

• **Interactions**: May interact with anticoagulant drugs, aspirin, antiplatelet drugs, statins, and drugs used to treat high blood pressure.

FOODS THAT TRANSFORM

"When food is bad, medicine does not work. When food is good, medicine is not necessary" (Ayurvedic proverb)

Throughout history, our diet has undergone profoundly radical changes, sharply diverging from the habits of our ancestors. Millions of years ago, early humans shaped their diet around what they could gather or hunt, relying on fresh and raw foods provided by their environment. The emergence of agriculture and livestock farming marked the beginning of a new era of human nutrition, further accelerated by the Industrial Revolution. However, it is important to recognize that while our dietary habits have evolved drastically, our genetics have remained virtually unchanged.

Over time, foods such as dairy products, grains, refined sugars, and vegetable oils were introduced, alongside the rise of intensive meat production. These innovations have made meals more accessible and convenient, yet they have also led to significant changes in nutritional composition. Furthermore, advances in food preservation and culinary techniques gave rise to new methods of storage and preparation, which inevitably impacted food quality.

In recent years, an alarming trend has surfaced: modern diets have become dominated by ultra-processed foods, contributing to the widespread increase in chronic illnesses. Conditions such as obesity, type 2 diabetes, hypertension, and a variety of cardiovascular and digestive disorders have all been closely linked to this dietary shift. Why is this happening? Primarily because ultra-processed foods are heavily laden with refined carbohydrates, unhealthy fats, added sugars, chemical additives, and low-quality vegetable oils. Even meats and other animal products from intensive farming systems are often filled with substances harmful to health. These processed foods have largely replaced traditional diets, which were built on fresh and natural ingredients, disrupting the equilibrium that once fostered optimal well-being among our ancestors.

Nonetheless, there is hope for reversing this trend: small yet thoughtful changes to our eating habits can have a significant impact on our health. Returning to a balanced, nutrient-rich way of eating, centered on fresh, whole foods, is essential for establishing a strong foundation for wellness. Integrating fruits, vegetables, root vegetables, legumes, nuts, and seeds into the diet is a powerful step toward revitalizing the way we nourish ourselves. Despite this, one major challenge persists: the consumption of these natural, unprocessed foods remains astonishingly low in many parts of the world.

Choosing a lifestyle rooted in mindful eating not only helps prevent diseases associated with poor dietary habits but also rejuvenates the body and mind. By prioritizing real, wholesome foods and cutting back on ultra-processed options, we can cultivate a healthier, more balanced, and fulfilling life. Now is the time to rediscover the transformative power of a healthy diet– not as a form of restriction, but as an act of self-care. Your health deserves that commitment!

Understanding the Link Between Nutrition and Health

How often have you asked yourself if what you eat truly supports your well-being? The relationship between nutrition and health is far deeper than we commonly realize. Understanding which foods promote wellness and which ones to avoid, tailored to your specific needs, is a powerful step toward improving your quality of life. This isn't a new concept; it has been examined and revered for centuries. Since ancient times, cultures around the world have recognized the therapeutic value of nutrition as a means to heal, strengthen, and sustain the body, leaving us a profound legacy of wisdom.

Traditional medical systems–such as Traditional Chinese Medicine, the practices of ancient Egypt, Greece, and Rome, Ayurveda in India, and indigenous healing methods across the

Americas—delved into the restorative potential of natural foods. These practices emphasized the idea that food does much more than nourish; it can protect, alleviate discomfort, and even heal the body.

For many years, these age-old principles were often dismissed by conventional medicine as unscientific. Yet, modern research has gradually confirmed what our ancestors intuitively understood: the foods we eat directly affect not only our physical health but also our emotional well-being. Today, scientific studies continue to uncover compounds in food with therapeutic properties that help prevent diseases, reduce symptoms, and promote overall health.

Researchers have spent decades analyzing how certain foods strengthen the body and protect against chronic illnesses, identifying dietary patterns in populations with low disease rates that differ significantly from those in less healthy communities. These studies reveal the decisive role specific nutrients play in promoting vitality and longevity, with certain foods offering unique benefits such as anti-inflammatory properties to manage joint pain and chronic discomfort, antimicrobial effects to bolster immune defenses, anticoagulant actions to support cardiovascular health, antihypertensive abilities to regulate blood pressure, and mood-enhancing compounds that alleviate anxiety while fostering emotional resilience.

What you choose to eat influences not only your daily energy but also your capacity to recover, fend off illness, and pursue a fulfilling life. On the flip side, a poor diet or reliance on unhealthy foods can exacerbate health problems, intensify symptoms, and undermine overall well-being.

The encouraging part? Every day offers the chance to make dietary choices that lead to better health. While external factors like pollution or environmental changes may remain out of your control, your diet is a fundamental tool for self-care. Each ingredient on your plate carries the potential to positively impact both your physical and mental health.

Learning which foods are best for your unique needs—and

understanding which ones may harm your health–can empower you to find balance and achieve a healthier, more vibrant lifestyle. Nutrition, humanity's earliest form of medicine, is not just a pathway to wellness but also a connection to our roots, equipping us for a future filled with possibilities.

I invite you to explore how nutrition can become your strongest ally in easing ailments, building resilience, and fostering happiness. Are you ready to embrace this journey of discovery and transformation? Your well-being is within your control, and every meal is a chance to create a life of greater health and vitality. Start today: Nourish your body, refresh your mind, and live fully.

Foods that Heal According to TCM

Traditional Chinese Medicine (TCM) emphasizes the value of certain foods that can be remarkably effective in alleviating and improving the symptoms of varicose veins. These foods, renowned for their anti-inflammatory properties, not only help reduce venous dilation but also provide relief from associated discomfort. They are rich in fiber and loaded with essential nutrients, including bioflavonoids, vitamins A, B, C, and E, as well as potassium and minerals like zinc. Together, these nutrients play a crucial role in strengthening the walls of veins and promoting overall vascular health.

It's also essential to highlight the role of proper hydration. Drinking at least one and a half liters of water daily (approximately six glasses) is vital for supporting healthy blood circulation, which is especially important for managing this condition.

Below is an alphabetical list of foods recommended for maintaining healthy veins. Explore these options and enhance your well-being with every bite!

Apricot (Prunus armeniaca)

Ingredients: 50 g apricot kernels and 50 g non-glutinous round rice.

Preparation: Grind the kernels and soak them in water for 2 hours. Extract the juice and boil it in 1.5 liters of water until it's reduced to half a liter. Add the rice and prepare a soup. Drink it twice a day.

Precautions: According to Traditional Chinese Medicine (TCM), due to its hot nature, excessive consumption of apricots may cause ulcerations of a hot nature, potentially leading to blindness and alopecia. Therefore, consume only the recommended amount. People with chronic internal heat should avoid it. The apricot kernel contains amygdalin, which converts into hydrocyanic acid when ingested, a highly toxic substance, so it should not be consumed in excess.

Fig (Ficus carica)

Ingredients: 2 fresh, unripe figs.

Preparation: Consume figs in the morning and evening.

Precautions: According to TCM, fresh figs have laxative properties, so people with loose or liquid stools should not consume them.

Adzuki Bean (Phaseolus angularis)

Ingredients: 60 g of adzuki beans and pork casing.

Preparation: Boil everything on low heat until well-cooked. Drink this broth for 4 to 6 days.

Precautions: According to TCM, adzuki beans are diuretic, so excessive consumption may cause fluid and weight loss. People who urinate frequently and in large quantities should consume them with caution.

Kiwi (Actinidia chinensis)

Ingredients: 200 g of fresh kiwi.

Preparation: Consume peeled and crushed kiwi twice daily, in the morning and at night.

Precautions: According to TCM, kiwi can cause diarrhea if consumed in excess due to its cold nature. Therefore, it should not be consumed in large quantities, especially by people prone to diarrhea or sensitive stomach issues.

Tofu

Ingredients: half a slice of tofu, 1 teaspoon of sugar, and water.

Preparation: Place the tofu and sugar in a pot and add water to cover the tofu. Bring to a boil and then reduce the heat, maintaining it for 5 minutes. Turn off the heat and remove the tofu. Consume this preparation on an empty stomach in the morning.

Other Foods That Will Help You

In addition to those mentioned earlier, incorporating the following foods into your diet can offer significant benefits for the health of your veins and help alleviate the discomfort caused by varicose veins:

• **Garlic**: Celebrated for its potent anti-inflammatory and decongestant properties, garlic enhances circulation and helps prevent the buildup of fatty plaques in your veins. To maximize its benefits, it is recommended to consume one clove of garlic on an empty stomach with a glass of water. You can also effortlessly incorporate it into your favorite dishes, enriching both the flavor and the health of your venous system.

• **Fruits and vegetables that promote circulation**: Boost your intake of fruits and vegetables that improve blood flow, such as pineapple, blackberries, strawberries, cherries, blueberries, watermelon, peaches, celery, and carrots. These delicious options also serve as excellent allies in strengthening your vascular health.

- **Vitamin C sources**: Fruits rich in vitamin C, such as oranges, lemons, grapefruits, kiwis, guavas, mangoes, and papayas, play a vital role in strengthening veins and capillaries, preventing fat buildup in the blood, and supporting better circulation. Vitamin C can also be found in vegetables like bell peppers, tomatoes, Brussels sprouts, and parsley. However, if you suffer from hemorrhoids, consider consuming citrus fruits in moderation, as excessive intake may cause irritation.

- **Foods rich in antioxidants**: Antioxidants are crucial for preventing the weakening and degradation of venous walls. Excellent sources include avocados, raspberries, grapes, tomatoes, onions, spinach, and cabbage.

- **Potassium sources**: Potassium-rich foods, such as bananas, avocados, and brewer's yeast, help the body eliminate excess fluids, reducing inflammation and preventing the development of edema commonly associated with varicose veins.

- **Turmeric**: This versatile spice is known for its anti-inflammatory and anticoagulant properties, which support improved blood flow. Adding turmeric to your meals is an easy way to take advantage of its many natural benefits.

- **Onions**: Onions are particularly effective for preventing the formation of clots in veins and arteries, making them an excellent choice for individuals dealing with varicose veins. Enjoy them raw, boiled, or roasted, and incorporate them into your favorite recipes effortlessly.

Other Remedies for Topical Use

Caring for your legs externally can be just as important as addressing their needs internally. Below, you'll find easy-to-prepare natural remedies specifically designed to stimulate circulation, reduce swelling, and alleviate the discomfort caused by varicose veins:

- **Aloe Vera with Apple Cider Vinegar**: Harness the

soothing properties of aloe vera and the stimulating benefits of apple cider vinegar. Blend fresh aloe vera pulp with apple cider vinegar until you create a smooth, consistent mixture. Gently apply the mixture to your legs using upward, circular massages to promote healthy venous return. Once applied, elevate your legs and allow the mixture to absorb into your skin. Repeat this process daily for noticeable relief.

• **Apple Cider Vinegar Compresses**: Elevating your legs is essential to enhancing circulation. Soak a clean cloth in apple cider vinegar and place it gently on the affected areas, avoiding pressure on inflamed veins. This simple remedy helps reduce inflammation and alleviates feelings of heaviness in the legs, leaving them refreshed and revitalized.

• **Aloe Vera, Apple Cider Vinegar, and Carrot Paste**: Create a powerful, natural paste by blending aloe vera gel, three tablespoons of apple cider vinegar, and one carrot until smooth. Apply the paste directly to the areas with varicose veins and let it sit for 30 minutes before rinsing thoroughly with cool water. This remedy combines the regenerative properties of aloe vera, the revitalizing effects of apple cider vinegar, and the antioxidant-rich nutrients of carrots.

• **Relaxing Soaking Baths**: For instant relief, immerse your legs in a soothing bath. Fill a bucket with warm water, add one cup of apple cider vinegar, and a tablespoon of sea salt. Soak your legs for 20 minutes, allowing the warm solution to ease heavy sensations and reduce inflammation.

By incorporating these simple yet effective remedies into your daily routine, you can significantly improve the health of your legs. Show them the extra care they need and deserve!

Recommended Food and Beverages

If you struggle with varicose veins or circulation issues, maintaining a mindful diet is essential. Below is a curated selection of foods and beverages that can significantly enhance vein health, strengthen their structure, and promote more efficient circulation.

• **Fiber-rich foods**: First, it is advisable to include fiber-rich foods in your diet. Fiber helps prevent constipation, which can add pressure to the veins and worsen varicose veins. Fruits, vegetables, legumes, whole grains, and nuts are excellent sources of fiber. Additionally, fiber promotes healthy digestion and helps maintain a proper weight, which is essential for reducing pressure on veins.

• **Antioxidant-rich foods**: Antioxidant-rich foods are also recommended to help strengthen blood vessels and reduce inflammation. Brightly colored fruits and vegetables, such as berries, grapes, citrus fruits, spinach, and tomatoes, are abundant in antioxidants. These foods are also rich in vitamin C, essential for collagen formation and maintaining the structure of blood vessels.

• **Foods rich in vitamin E**: Foods rich in vitamin E also benefit vascular health. Vitamin E acts as an antioxidant, helping to prevent the formation of blood clots. Natural sources of vitamin E include nuts, seeds, avocados, and olive oil.

• **Omega-3**: Furthermore, foods rich in omega-3 fatty acids should be included in the diet. These fatty acids have anti-inflammatory properties and can help improve blood circulation. Fatty fish, such as salmon, tuna, and sardines, are excellent sources of omega-3. They can also be found in chia seeds, walnuts, and flaxseed oil.

• **Foods rich in flavonoids**: Consuming foods rich in flavonoids may also benefit varicose veins. Flavonoids are plant compounds that help strengthen blood vessels and improve circulation. Some foods rich in flavonoids include berries, citrus fruits, green tea, cocoa, onions, and garlic.

• **Water**: Regarding beverages, staying hydrated and drinking enough water throughout the day is essential. Adequate hydration helps maintain good blood circulation and prevents fluid retention. Additionally, you can incorporate herbal infusions such as chamomile, peppermint, or witch hazel, which possess anti-inflammatory properties and can help alleviate the symptoms of varicose veins.

Foods and Beverages to Limit or Avoid

If you're living with varicose veins, certain foods and drinks can worsen symptoms and heighten discomfort. While diet alone isn't a definitive cure, it plays a vital role in managing the condition and preventing it from getting worse. Reducing or avoiding these items can help minimize inflammation, boost circulation, and ease associated discomfort. Your body will thank you for it!

- **Foods high in sodium**: Excessive sodium intake can lead to fluid retention and swelling, which can exacerbate the appearance and symptoms of varicose veins. Avoid reducing your intake of processed foods, such as sausages, fast food, and canned soups, which are often high in sodium.

- **Saturated and trans fats**: Limit saturated and trans fats because they can clog arteries and impede blood circulation, which increases pressure in the veins and worsens varicose veins. Avoid fried foods, high-fat processed foods, and full-fat dairy products.

- **Refined sugars and simple carbohydrates**: Reduce your consumption of refined sugars and simple carbohydrates. These can elevate blood sugar levels, contributing to inflammation and damage to blood vessel walls. Limiting sweets, cakes, cookies, soft drinks, and sugary juices is the best approach.

- **Alcohol**: Avoid excessive alcohol consumption, as alcohol can dilate blood vessels and increase pressure in the veins, worsening the symptoms and appearance of varicose veins. Alcohol can also dehydrate the body and hinder blood circulation.

- **Caffeine**: Moderate your caffeine intake. Coffee and tea contain caffeine, which can act as vasoconstrictors, narrowing blood vessels and impeding blood circulation. Consider alternatives like herbal teas or water.

Key Nutritional Tips for Healthy Veins

In addition to including specific foods that promote vein health, adopting certain dietary habits and making thoughtful nutritional choices can significantly aid in managing varicose veins. These recommendations not only improve circulation and reduce inflammation but also support an overall healthier lifestyle. Follow these tips to enhance your diet's benefits and feel your best every day.

- **Fiber intake**: Fiber is essential for improving circulation and preventing constipation, which can worsen varicose vein symptoms. Be sure to include fiber-rich foods in your diet, such as fruits, vegetables, legumes, whole grains, and nuts.

- **Antioxidants**: Antioxidants help reduce inflammation and oxidative damage to blood vessels. Include foods rich in antioxidants in your diet, such as brightly colored fruits and vegetables like blueberries, strawberries, oranges, spinach, and broccoli.

- **Omega-3 fatty acids**: Omega-3 fatty acids have anti-inflammatory properties and contribute to improved cardiovascular health. You can find them in fatty fish such as salmon, mackerel, and sardines, as well as in chia seeds, walnuts, and olive oil.

- **Vitamin C**: Vitamin C is essential for collagen formation, which helps maintain the elasticity of blood vessels. Be sure to include foods rich in vitamin C in your diet, such as citrus fruits, kiwis, strawberries, peppers, and tomatoes.

- **Adequate hydration**: Drinking enough water is crucial for maintaining good blood circulation. Try to consume at least 8 glasses of water a day and avoid excessive consumption of diuretic beverages, such as coffee and alcohol, which can dehydrate you. Increase your water intake if it is summer or if you engage in sports. This will improve blood flow and help avoid constipation and hard stools, which can also worsen hemorrhoids if you suffer from them.

- **Salt reduction**: Consuming high amounts of salt can

contribute to fluid retention and worsen leg swelling. Limit your intake of processed foods and avoid adding extra salt to your meals.

• **Avoid inflammatory foods**: Some foods can increase inflammation and worsen the symptoms of varicose veins. Limit your consumption of processed foods, fried foods, saturated fats, refined sugars, and refined flour.

• **Avoid consuming extremely cold or hot foods and beverages**. They should be at room temperature.

• **Avoid large meals**. Instead, eat more frequently, smaller meals throughout the day, totaling 4 or 5.

• **Do not reuse the same cooking oil** more than once.

Cooking Techniques

Healthy cooking is essential for everyone, especially after the age of 40. Below are various cooking techniques along with their related health benefits and potential risks.

Healthier Ways of Cooking

• **Steaming**: Steaming is an excellent method for preserving nutrients, as it does not require the use of additional fats. It helps keep food tender and juicy while being a gentle cooking technique that does not contribute to the formation of harmful compounds.

• **Oven roasting**: Oven roasting is a healthy option that does not require added oils. Foods like vegetables, fish, and chicken can be roasted in the oven to create nutritious and flavorful meals.

• **Light sautéing**: This method involves quickly cooking food over high heat with a small amount of healthy oil, such as olive or coconut oil. Light sautéing helps maintain the food's texture and nutrients while cooking it efficiently.

• **Boiling**: Boiling is a healthy cooking method, particularly for vegetables. It preserves nutrients and creates a tender texture. However, it is crucial to avoid overcooking to minimize nutrient loss.

• **Baking**: Baking is an excellent way to prepare food without the need for added oils. Foods like fish, poultry, vegetables, and whole grains can be baked for healthy and flavorful dishes.

Less Healthy Ways of Cooking

• **Frying**: Frying involves submerging food in hot oil, which significantly increases its saturated fat and calorie content. Additionally, frying at high temperatures can produce harmful compounds that pose health risks.

• **Breading and battering**: Coating food in breading or batter increases its calorie and fat content. These coatings can absorb more oil during cooking, resulting in a less nutritious meal.

• **Creamy sauces and dressings**: Cream-based sauces and dressings often contain high levels of saturated fat and excess calories. These can contribute to inflammation and exacerbate pain.

• **Grilling at high temperatures**: Cooking food on the grill at high heat can generate harmful compounds, such as polycyclic aromatic hydrocarbons (PAHs) and heterocyclic amines (HCAs), which have been associated with an increased cancer risk. Additionally, grilled meats can produce inflammatory substances.

Remember, the way you cook food significantly impacts its nutritional value and its overall effects on your health. Choosing healthy cooking methods ensures you maximize the benefits of your meals while reducing potential negative effects.

Varicose Veins Support: Easy and Tasty Recipes

Discover a selection of quick, simple, and flavorful recipes specially crafted to promote vein health and improve circulation. Taking care of yourself has never been so enjoyable!

Breakfast Options

1. Fruit and vegetable smoothie: Blend one cup of spinach, half a banana, half a cup of blueberries, one tablespoon of chia seeds, and water. Blend until smooth and enjoy.

2. Avocado toast: Spread fresh avocado on a slice of whole wheat bread. You can add tomato, cucumber, or hard-boiled egg for more flavor and nutrients.

3. Yogurt with granola and fruit: Combine plain low-fat yogurt with your favorite granola and add some fresh fruit, such as strawberries or blueberries.

4. Oatmeal with fruit: Prepare a bowl of cooked oatmeal and add banana slices, blueberries, or any other fruit you choose. You can add a tablespoon of flax or chia seeds for additional fiber.

5. Egg white omelet with spinach: Mix egg whites with chopped spinach and cook over medium heat until set. Serve with a slice of whole wheat bread or a corn tortilla.

6. Oatmeal banana pancakes: Mix ground oats, ripe bananas, egg whites, and ground cinnamon. Cook the mixture in a non-stick pan until golden brown on both sides.

7. Rye toast with avocado and salmon: Toast slices of rye bread and spread them with mashed avocado. Add some slices of smoked salmon and a little lemon juice for a touch of freshness.

8. Beet and berry smoothie: Blend cooked beets, berries such as strawberries and raspberries, plain yogurt, and a splash of orange juice until smooth, then enjoy.

9. Spinach and feta cheese omelet: Beat eggs with chopped spinach and crumbled feta cheese. Cook the mixture in a non-stick frying pan until it sets. Serve with a fresh salad.

Lunch Creations

1. Spinach and salmon salad: Combine fresh spinach with grilled salmon chunks. Add cucumber slices, cherry tomatoes, and sunflower seeds. Dress with olive oil and lemon juice.

2. Quinoa with roasted vegetables: Cook quinoa according to package directions and let it cool. Toss quinoa with roasted vegetables such as carrots, zucchini, and peppers. Dress with lemon vinaigrette.

3. Grilled chicken breast with avocado salad: Grill chicken breasts and serve them with a salad of avocado, tomato, cucumber, and mixed greens. Dress the salad with a light vinaigrette.

4. Vegetable and hummus wraps: Fill whole wheat tortillas with hummus, spinach, cucumber, tomato, and roasted peppers. Wrap the ingredients together and enjoy a quick and nutritious lunch.

5. Lentil and vegetable soup: Cook lentils in vegetable broth and add carrots, celery, onion, and spinach–season with herbs and spices to taste. Serve hot with a slice of whole-wheat bread.

6. Chickpea and avocado salad: Combine cooked chickpeas, diced avocado, cherry tomatoes, red onion, and fresh cilantro. Dress with olive oil, lime juice, and salt. For a heartier salad, add leafy greens.

7. Baked salmon with asparagus: Place salmon fillets in a baking dish and add fresh asparagus. Drizzle with olive oil, lemon juice, salt, and pepper. Bake at 180°C until the salmon is cooked and the asparagus is tender.

8. Quinoa salad with grilled chicken: Mix cooked quinoa with pieces of grilled chicken breast. Add spinach, tomato, cucumber, avocado, and olives. Dress with a lemon vinaigrette and fresh herbs.

9. Vegetable stir-fry with tofu: Sauté a variety of vegetables such as broccoli, carrots, peppers, and mushrooms in a skillet with olive oil. Add tofu cubes and season with low-sodium soy sauce.

10. Chickpea and tuna salad: Combine cooked chickpeas, canned tuna, tomato, cucumber, red onion, and olives in a salad bowl. Dress with olive oil, balsamic vinegar, salt, and pepper.

11. Vegetable soup with quinoa: Cook a variety of vegetables such as carrots, zucchini, peppers, and spinach in vegetable broth. Add cooked quinoa and season with herbs and spices to taste.

12. Chicken and avocado salad: Combine cooked chicken pieces, avocado, tomato, lettuce, corn, and cilantro in a salad bowl–dress with Greek yogurt, lime juice, minced garlic, salt, and pepper.

13. Chickpea salad with avocado and egg: Combine cooked chickpeas, diced avocado, chopped hard-boiled egg, cherry tomatoes, and greens. Dress with a honey mustard vinaigrette.

14. Lettuce rolls with chicken and vegetables: Stuff lettuce leaves with shredded cooked chicken, shredded carrots, julienned cucumber, and bell pepper strips. For more flavor, add yogurt sauce or hummus.

15. Baked fish with steamed vegetables: Place fish fillets, such as tilapia or hake, on a baking sheet. Add a variety of steamed vegetables, such as broccoli, carrots, and zucchini.

Sprinkle with lemon juice and fresh herbs before baking.

16. Chicken salad with walnuts and grapes: Combine cooked chicken, chopped walnuts, halved grapes, sliced celery, and greens. Dress with a honey mustard vinaigrette.

17. Tomato and red lentil soup: Cook red lentils with vegetable broth and add crushed tomatoes, carrots, onion, and spices such as cumin and sweet paprika. Serve hot with a slice of whole wheat bread.

18. Quinoa salad with falafel: Mix cooked quinoa with baked falafel, cucumber, tomato, red onion, and greens. Dress with a lemon vinaigrette and fresh herbs.

Snacks

1. Carrot sticks and hummus: Cut carrots into sticks and serve them with homemade or store-bought hummus. Hummus is rich in fiber and protein.

2. Apple slices with almond butter: Slice an apple and spread almond butter on each piece. Almonds contain vitamin E, which can help improve blood vessel health.

3. Ham and spinach rolls: Wrap slices of lean ham around fresh spinach leaves. This snack is low in calories and rich in iron and vitamin C.

4. Berry smoothie: Blend frozen berries (strawberries, raspberries, blueberries) with low-fat yogurt or plant-based milk. You can add a spoonful of nuts or seeds for an extra boost of nutrients.

5. Cucumber slices with Greek yogurt: Slice cucumbers and serve with a dollop of unsweetened Greek yogurt. Cucumber contains water and fiber, which can help with blood circulation.

6. Nut and dried fruit bars: Mix chopped nuts, dried fruits such as dates or dried plums, sunflower seeds, and shredded coconut. Form into small bars and refrigerate. These are practical and nutritious on-the-go options.

7. Turkey and avocado rolls: Slice low-sodium turkey and add a tablespoon of avocado to each slice. Roll them up and secure them with a toothpick. These are a quick, low-fat option to enjoy between meals.

8. Baked kale chips: Cut kale leaves into pieces, drizzle with olive oil, and season with salt and pepper. Bake at a low temperature until crispy.

9. Green smoothie: Blend spinach, pineapple, banana, a handful of mint leaves, and a little water until smooth and refreshing. Add a bit of ginger for an extra touch of flavor.

Dinner Ideas

1. Spinach and salmon salad: Combine fresh spinach with grilled salmon, and add walnuts, chia seeds, and a lemon vinaigrette dressing for a nutritious meal rich in omega-3 fatty acids.

2. Grilled chicken with steamed vegetables: Grill chicken breasts and serve with various steamed vegetables, such as broccoli, carrots, and zucchini–season with herbs and spices for added flavor.

3. Quinoa with sautéed vegetables: Cook quinoa and mix it with sautéed vegetables, such as peppers, onions, mushrooms, and spinach. Add a little olive oil and lemon juice to enhance the flavor.

4. Lentil soup: Prepare a delicious lentil soup with vegetables such as carrots, celery, and tomatoes. Lentils are rich in fiber and protein and can help promote good blood circulation.

5. Baked fish with asparagus: Bake fish fillets, such as salmon or trout, along with fresh asparagus. Sprinkle with lemon, garlic, and olive oil for a tasty and nutritious dish.

6. Beet and orange salad: Combine grated beets, orange slices, spinach leaves, and walnuts. Dress with a light balsamic vinegar and olive oil dressing.

7. Turkey tacos with avocado: Grill turkey breasts and cut them into thin strips. Fill whole wheat tortillas with the turkey, avocado slices, tomato, and cilantro. Serve with a low-fat yogurt sauce.

8. Eggplants stuffed with quinoa and vegetables: Cut eggplants in half and scoop out some of the flesh. Fill them with a mixture of cooked quinoa, chopped vegetables such as peppers and onions, and low-fat cheese. Bake until tender and golden brown.

9. Pumpkin soup: Cook pumpkin chunks with vegetable broth, onion, and garlic. Once cooked, blend until smooth. To enhance the flavor, add spices such as nutmeg and cinnamon.

10. Lemon chicken breasts with asparagus: Grill chicken breasts with lemon juice, garlic, and fresh herbs. Serve with steamed or grilled asparagus for a light and nutritious dinner.

11. Baked salmon with roasted vegetables: Place salmon fillets on a baking sheet and add a mixture of carrots, zucchini, cherry tomatoes, and peppers. Drizzle with olive oil, herbs, and spices, and bake until the salmon is tender and the vegetables are golden brown.

12. Chickpea salad: Combine cooked chickpeas with cucumber, tomato, red onion, and sliced black olives. Dress with lemon juice, olive oil, and fresh herbs such as parsley or cilantro. You can add low-fat feta cheese if desired.

13. Turkey curry with brown rice: Sauté turkey breast pieces with onion, garlic, and spices. Add coconut milk and simmer until the meat is tender. Serve over cooked brown rice.

14. Quinoa and avocado salad: Mix cooked quinoa with diced avocado, cherry tomatoes, cucumber, cilantro, and lime juice. Dress with olive oil, salt, and pepper to taste. This salad is rich in fiber and healthy fats.

15. Lettuce rolls with teriyaki chicken: Cook chicken breast strips with low-sodium teriyaki sauce. Wrap chicken strips in lettuce leaves and add shredded carrot, green onion, and cilantro. Serve with low-sodium soy sauce for dipping.

16. Peppers stuffed with quinoa and vegetables: Cut the peppers in half and remove the seeds. Fill them with a mixture of cooked quinoa, chopped vegetables such as zucchini, spinach, mushrooms, and low-fat cheese. Bake until the peppers are tender and the cheese is melted.

17. Broccoli and cheese soup: Cook broccoli pieces with vegetable broth, onion, and garlic until tender. Then, blend the mixture until smooth. Add low-fat cheddar cheese and stir until melted. Season to taste and serve hot.

18. Smoked salmon and avocado salad: Combine lettuce leaves, spinach, smoked salmon strips, diced avocado, and cucumber slices. Dress with a light lemon-mustard vinaigrette.

19. Baked chicken with vegetables and papillote: Place chicken breasts on aluminum foil or parchment paper. Add vegetables such as carrots, zucchini, and peppers–season with herbs, spices, and a drizzle of olive oil. Close the foil into a packet and bake until the chicken is cooked and the vegetables are tender.

20. Fish tacos with yogurt sauce: Marinate white fish fillets in lime juice, garlic, and spices. Grill or bake until tender. Then, place the fillets in corn tortillas and add a yogurt sauce with lime, cilantro, and chopped cucumber.

Remember to adjust the recipes according to your preferences and dietary needs. I hope you enjoy these healthy options for your meals!

JUICES & SMOOTHIES

"Enjoy your good health; only those who are well are young" (Voltaire)

Raw foods, often referred to as "living" foods, are an exceptional source of vitamins, minerals, fiber, trace elements, enzymes, and other vital compounds that support overall health. Incorporating these nutrient-rich foods into your daily diet not only aids in disease prevention but also alleviates symptoms of various health conditions, slows down the aging process, balances gut flora, and enhances energy levels and vitality.

While salads, whole fruits, and nuts are excellent raw food options, one of the easiest and most convenient ways to ensure regular intake is by preparing homemade juices, smoothies, and shakes. These beverages serve as a delicious and practical alternative for individuals who may not enjoy consuming fruits and vegetables directly, making it easier to include these essential nutrients in their diet.

In today's world, where ultra-processed foods and toxins have become increasingly prevalent, the need for natural, nutrient-dense foods is more crucial than ever. Raw foods play a vital role in supporting detoxification, maintaining health, and restoring balance to the body.

Many people tend to prepare their juices and smoothies using only fruits, often overlooking the incredible health benefits vegetables and leafy greens provide. Adding these to your recipes not only increases variety but also significantly boosts their nutritional value, enhancing their antioxidant, remineralizing, toning, and alkalizing properties. These qualities help maintain the body's balance, rejuvenate cells, and promote overall well-being. Additionally, vegetables and greens lower the glycemic index, improve satiety, and maximize the health benefits of these preparations.

However, it is crucial to understand that most store-bought juices are far from healthy options. These commercial products are often loaded with excessive added sugars, artificial sweeteners, preservatives, and harmful chemical additives. Furthermore, the pasteurization processes used during production strip away essential vitamins and enzymes, rendering them nutritionally deficient. The high level of refinement also removes fiber, a vital component of whole foods. In many cases, these juices contain only minimal amounts of actual fruit, making them highly processed and lacking true nutritional value.

One major concern with many juices and smoothies is their high glycemic index, which can cause blood sugar spikes, lead to weight gain, and contribute to long-term metabolic imbalances. To truly enjoy healthy and nourishing beverages, the best approach is to prepare them at home using fresh, natural, and high-quality ingredients. Homemade juices and smoothies are packed with nutrients that provide genuine benefits for your body and overall well-being.

Incorporating fresh juices made from fruits, vegetables, and leafy greens into your daily routine is an excellent practice for maintaining a healthy and energetic body. With endless combinations to explore, you can enjoy not only flavorful and refreshing options but also targeted health benefits, such as relief from conditions like arthritis, thanks to essential nutrients that support wellness. Making this a part of your everyday life can transform your health, boost your energy, and elevate your quality of life. Try it for yourself and feel the difference!

Juices: Unleash Their Power

Incorporating smoothies or shakes into your diet can be a fantastic way to boost your health. Below are some of their most significant benefits:

- **Compliance with Recommended Fruit and Vegetable**

Intake: Smoothies and shakes offer a practical and enjoyable way to meet the daily recommendation of five servings of fruits and vegetables. They provide a diverse range of essential nutrients that support optimal health and overall well-being.

• **Easy Assimilation and Digestion:** As liquid meals, smoothies and shakes are gentler on the digestive system and allow for quicker nutrient absorption. They are especially beneficial for individuals with digestive sensitivities or challenges.

• **Vitamin and Mineral Powerhouse:** Made from fresh fruits and vegetables, smoothies and shakes are rich sources of essential vitamins and minerals that promote the proper functioning of the body.

• **Detoxification and Cleansing:** Ingredients like leafy greens and natural antioxidants help flush out toxins, enhance cell health, and support effective internal cleansing.

• **Balancing Body pH:** By incorporating alkaline foods, smoothies and shakes play a key role in stabilizing the body's pH levels, aiding disease prevention and improving overall wellness.

• **Reduction of Inflammation:** Anti-inflammatory additions such as turmeric, ginger, and leafy greens can help minimize inflammation, fostering better health and increased comfort.

• **A Balanced Meal Replacement:** When combined with protein, healthy fats, and complex carbohydrates, smoothies become a nourishing and balanced meal replacement. They provide sustained energy and promote fullness throughout the day.

• **Supports Weight Management:** With their low-calorie yet nutrient-dense profiles, smoothies and shakes encourage healthy eating habits. They help manage appetite and support maintaining or achieving an ideal weight.

- **Enhances Skin Health**: Packed with skin-friendly vitamins like A and C from fresh ingredients, smoothies and shakes contribute to hydrated, radiant, and healthy skin.

- **Slows Cellular Aging**: The antioxidants in smoothie ingredients combat oxidative damage, protect cells, and help maintain a youthful appearance.

- **Boosts Energy and Vitality**: Smoothies made with superfoods provide a steady energy boost, helping you stay active, energized, and revitalized throughout the day.

In conclusion, smoothies and shakes are a nutritious, convenient, and versatile addition to your diet. Not only do they make it easier to meet your daily fruit and vegetable intake, but they also offer a wide array of health benefits. Packed with essential nutrients, they support overall well-being —all while being refreshing, delicious, and easy to enjoy.

Homemade vs. Commercial Juices

Nowadays, identifying which foods truly benefit our health can be quite challenging. Supermarkets are overflowing with an extensive range of options, flaunting attractive packaging and clever designs that promise to be natural and healthy. While advertising and packaging often catch our attention, are we genuinely purchasing natural beverages made from fruits and vegetables? Do you know the key differences between homemade juices and industrial products? Are packaged products really as nutritious as they claim to be? Taking a few moments to carefully read ingredient labels and analyze their composition may uncover some surprising truths.

A few years ago, international regulations were established to define the standards that every fruit-based beverage must meet, specifying precise characteristics for each type of product. Below, we'll explore these distinctions and delve into the essential differences.

- **Fruit Juice**

Fruit juice is derived from fresh, chilled, or frozen fruits without undergoing any fermentation. It may contain separately extracted pulp and, in some cases, be blended with juice from various fruits. Labels are required to specify the composition in descending order, including the exact percentage of each fruit.

To prolong shelf life and eliminate the need for refrigeration, fruit juice is typically sterilized or pasteurized. Unfortunately, these processes result in significant nutrient loss, particularly impacting essential vitamins and enzymes. Moreover, the juice lacks the natural fiber found in whole fruits.

• Juice from Concentrates

Juice from concentrates is created by reconstituting dehydrated juice concentrates with water. Concentrates are produced by extracting natural juice through evaporation or other physical methods. During reconstitution, manufacturers may add aromas or pulp from similar fruits to partially restore flavor.

Though widely consumed, these juices suffer nutrient losses during production, including enzymes, vitamins, minerals, and the valuable fiber that characterizes natural fruit.

• Dehydrated or Powdered Fruit Juice

This product is manufactured by removing water from fruit to create a dry powder, which can later be rehydrated or sold in its dehydrated state. However, the dehydration process significantly diminishes its nutritional value, leading to the loss of enzymes, vitamins, minerals, and natural fiber.

• Fruit Nectar

Fruit nectar differs from pure juice as it is made using fruit concentrate, water, and added sugars or sweeteners. Its nutritional value is considerably lower compared to natural fruit juices due to its inclusion of artificial additives to enhance flavor, color, or shelf life.

• Juice-Based Drinks

These beverages typically combine various fruits but contain minimal actual fruit juice. Often, they lack the essential nutrients derived from fruits, consisting largely of water, artificial aromas, colorings, and sweeteners.

• Milk-Infused Juice Drinks

Milk-infused juice drinks include fruit juice, often from concentrates, in very small proportions. They are mixed with milk, water, flavorings, and other ingredients. These beverages are not considered true juices, and any nutrients present are artificially added during manufacturing to compensate for losses incurred during processing.

• Vegetable and/or Greens Juice

Vegetable and greens juices are extracted from vegetables using specialized industrial methods, often with added pulp or pureed ingredients. They may also blend various vegetables to create balanced or palatable flavors.

To extend shelf life and eliminate refrigeration requirements, these juices undergo pasteurization or sterilization, which unfortunately reduces essential nutrients, including vitamins and phytonutrients. Additionally, they lack the natural fiber of whole vegetables and may include preservatives, salt, or flavor enhancers that compromise their nutritional profile.

• Commercial Smoothies

Commercial smoothies are typically prepared by blending fruits, vegetables, and greens–often using purees or concentrates–with water, milk, plant-based beverages, or similar liquids. Their thicker texture comes from a higher proportion of pulp or fiber-rich components.

To enhance taste, appearance, and shelf life, industrial smoothies usually contain added sugars, preservatives, colorings, and flavorings that alter their natural composition. Moreover, they undergo pasteurization or thermal sterilization to allow room-temperature storage, further degrading their original nutrients and reducing their overall nutritional quality.

Advantages of Homemade Juices

After discovering what commercial products truly contain, it becomes evident that making juices at home offers numerous advantages. Here are the key benefits:

- **Complete Control Over Ingredients**: Preparing your own

juices allows you to ensure the quality of the ingredients you use. There are no unnecessary additives, no preservatives, and–most importantly–no unpleasant surprises.

• **Variety and Creativity**: You have the freedom to choose your favorite fruits and vegetables, experiment with unique combinations, or incorporate fresh, seasonal produce. This not only provides a burst of delicious flavors but also boosts your intake of essential nutrients.

• **Authentic Aroma and Flavor**: Homemade juices retain the genuine aroma and taste of fresh fruits and vegetables. There's truly nothing like enjoying a freshly made juice packed with natural freshness.

• **Maximum Nutrient Retention**: Vitamins, minerals, enzymes, antioxidants, and other nutrients remain intact when you prepare juices at home, significantly enhancing their health benefits.

• **Premium Quality Ingredients**: Choosing fresh, seasonal produce at its peak ripeness ensures optimal flavor and exceptional nutritional value.

• **Seasonal Food Benefits**: Consuming fruits and vegetables that are in season supports sustainability, is more cost-effective, and often results in better taste and nutritional quality.

• **Total Customization**: Whether using a juicer or blender, you can adjust the consistency of your juice to your liking–whether you prefer a light, clear juice or a thicker, fiber-rich option.

• **Kid-Friendly Option**: Homemade juices are an excellent way to incorporate fruits and vegetables into children's diets, especially for picky eaters. With creative flavors and fun presentations, you can make juices irresistible for kids.

Making juices at home provides several compelling advantages: complete control over ingredients, enhanced nutrient retention, and the flexibility to tailor your drinks to your preferences. It's also a simple yet effective way to promote healthy eating for the whole family.

Possible Adverse Effects

If you suffer from **gastritis, colitis, SIBO, irritable bowel syndrome, or constipation,** it's essential to take certain precautions when preparing smoothies or juices. Following these recommendations will help you enjoy their benefits without worsening your symptoms:

- **Use a juicer instead of a blender**: For digestive health conditions, it's often better to use a juicer rather than a blender when making juices. Juicing removes most of the fiber from the ingredients, resulting in a smoother liquid that is gentler on your digestive system.

- **Moderate your fiber intake**: Although fiber is highly beneficial for overall health, excessive consumption can lead to gas, bloating, or constipation—especially for individuals with sensitive digestion. Be mindful of the fiber content in your smoothies by limiting ingredients like fruit pulp, seeds, and whole grains.

- **Introduce juices gradually**: If you're unsure how your body will react, start with small portions. This enables you to monitor their effects on your digestion and adjust the recipes to suit your specific needs.

- **Consume juices on an empty stomach**: Drinking juices on an empty stomach can maximize nutrient absorption and aid digestion. This approach minimizes the risk of digestive discomfort and helps you fully benefit from the juice's nutrients.

- **Tailor recipes to your personal needs**: Everyone's digestive system is unique, and responses to certain foods can vary greatly. Pay close attention to how your body reacts after consuming juices, and adapt ingredient combinations to best support your health and well-being.

When to Take Them

There are several effective ways to incorporate juices into your routine, depending on your goals and daily habits. Below are three recommended methods:

- **In the morning, on an empty stomach**: Begin your day with a carefully chosen juice recipe, consuming it before eating anything else. Drinking juice on an empty stomach enhances nutrient absorption and stimulates your digestive system, helping prepare it for the rest of the day.

- **On an empty stomach, before meals**: Enjoy a juice approximately 30 minutes before your main meals to maximize its benefits. This practice supports digestion and boosts nutrient absorption, promoting overall health and well-being.

- **Juice-based fasting**: Engage in a multi-day fast consisting exclusively of juices to achieve specific health objectives or to detoxify your body. Choose 2 to 3 recipes and consume them consistently throughout the day to stay nourished and energized.

Preparation Tips

Preparing fresh juices is an easy and nutritious way to make the most of the vitamins and minerals found in fruits and vegetables. To optimize the process and ensure safety, consider the following recommendations:

- **Choose organic ingredients**: Whenever possible, opt for organic fruits and vegetables. They provide cleaner, pesticide-free consumption and promote a healthier lifestyle.

- **Wash ingredients thoroughly**: Rinse all produce carefully to remove dirt, bacteria, and chemical residues. Trim any bruised, moldy, or damaged areas to prevent contamination.

- **Cut ingredients into smaller pieces**: Make blending easier by chopping fruits and vegetables into smaller, manageable chunks. This helps achieve a smoother texture and shortens preparation time.

- **Balance ingredients with low water content**: Fruits and vegetables with low water content, such as bananas and avocados, may require pre-mixing. Start with juicier ingredients to create a liquid base, then gradually add denser items for a cohesive blend.

- **Peel certain fruits appropriately**: Remove citrus rinds (like those from oranges and grapefruits), as their outer layers may contain toxins. However, keep the nutrient-rich white inner layer. Peel tropical fruits, such as papayas and kiwis, especially if they are grown in regions with less stringent chemical regulations.

- **Discard harmful seeds**: Remove seeds from apples, as they contain trace amounts of cyanide and are unsafe to consume. On the other hand, seeds from grapes, melons, lemons, and limes are safe and offer additional health benefits.

- **Incorporate stems and leaves mindfully**: Many stems and leaves are nutritious, but be cautious. Avoid toxic ones, such as carrot and rhubarb leaves, which can be harmful.

- **Drink your juice immediately**: Freshly prepared juice is best consumed right away to minimize nutrient loss and avoid oxidation. This ensures maximum freshness and health benefits.

- **Remove bitter celery leaves**: Bitter celery leaves can affect the flavor of your juice. Remove them before blending the stalks to create a more balanced and enjoyable taste.

Key Recommendations

Smoothies and shakes are an excellent, healthy alternative, but to get the most out of them, it's essential to keep certain aspects in mind. Below are some key recommendations:

- **Moderate fruit consumption**: Fruits are a fantastic source of nutrients but also contain fructose, a natural sugar that, when consumed excessively, can impact your health. Strive for balance by moderating your fruit intake throughout the day. Additionally, avoid eating fruits at night, as the body may metabolize them less efficiently during this time.

• **Choose seasonal fruits**: Seasonal fruits are often more nutrient-rich, flavorful, and cost-effective. By opting for fruits in season, you can enjoy their peak freshness and nutritional benefits while saving money.

• **Pick compatible combinations**: Not all fruits or ingredients blend well together. Research suitable pairings to create a smoothie or shake with balanced flavors and optimal nutritional value.

• **Use a moderate amount of ingredients**: The simplest smoothies are often the best. Avoid overloading them with excessive ingredients, which can lead to heavy textures or digestive discomfort. Stick to recommended recipes and be mindful of proportions.

• **Include leafy greens and vegetables**: Incorporate leafy greens, like spinach or kale, or vegetables, such as cucumber, to lower the glycemic index and boost your drink's nutrient profile. These additions make your smoothie both healthier and more satisfying.

• **Use natural sweeteners in moderation**: Enjoy the natural flavors of the ingredients, but if sweetening is necessary, choose options like raw honey or pure stevia. Use them sparingly to maintain a balanced nutritional profile.

• **Chew your drink**: Even liquid smoothies benefit from being "chewed." This simple habit stimulates the release of digestive enzymes, helping improve nutrient absorption and reducing discomfort like bloating or indigestion.

• **Store properly**: For the best results, consume smoothies or shakes fresh. If storing is needed, place them in a dark, airtight container in the refrigerator, or freeze individual portions for later use.

• **Make them fun and personalized**: Add an enjoyable twist by freezing smoothies in molds with fun shapes–an excellent way to turn a healthy drink into a delightful treat, especially for children.

These recommendations will help you make the most of your smoothies and shakes. While the recipes provided in this book are crafted to facilitate nutrient absorption, always remember that individual needs vary. Feel free to experiment with different combinations, tailor recipes to suit your tastes, and prioritize your health and well-being. Enjoy the journey to a healthier lifestyle!

Suggested Recipes

• **Fig, Orange, Grapefruit, and Lemon Juice:**
Ingredients: 2 figs, 1/2 small orange, 1/2 grapefruit, and 1/2 lemon.
Preparation: Wash the figs thoroughly. Peel the orange, grapefruit, and lemon, removing the white pith. Cut them into pieces and add them to the blender along with the figs.

• **Carrot and Spinach Juice:**
Ingredients: 6 to 7 carrots and a bunch of spinach.
Preparation: Clean the carrots and cut them into 5 to 7-centimeter-long strips. Blend the ingredients, starting and ending with the carrots. Consume 2 or 3 times a day.

• **Celery Juice:**
Ingredients: 5 celery stalks.
Preparation: Cut the celery into 5 to 7-centimeter-long strips, blend them, and consume them twice daily.

• **Celery and Carrot Juice:**
Ingredients: 4 celery stalks and 3 carrots.
Preparation: Cut the carrots and celery into 5 to 7-centimeter-long strips. Blend everything, starting and ending with the carrots. Consume 2 or 3 times a day.

- **Carrot, Apple, and Parsley Juice:**

Ingredients: 5 carrots, 1 apple, and 1 bunch of parsley.

Preparation: Clean the carrots and cut them into 5 to 7-centimeter-long strips. Cut the apple into thin slices. Blend half of the carrot pieces first, then the parsley, followed by the rest of the carrots. Finally, blend the apple. Mix well and drink 1 or 2 times a day.

- **Apple, Pear, and Ginger Juice:**

Ingredients: 2 apples, 1 pear, and 1 piece of ginger root (2 centimeters).

Preparation: Cut the apples, pear, and ginger into thin slices. Blend the ingredients, always starting and ending with the apples. Drink once a day.

- **Carrot, Celery, Spinach, and Parsley Juice:**

Ingredients: 4 carrots, 2 celery stalks, 1 bunch of spinach, and a handful of parsley.

Preparation: Clean the carrots and celery and cut them into 5 to 7-centimeter-long strips. Blend all ingredients. Drink 1 or 2 times daily (Note: This juice is rich in calcium).

- **Carrot, Apple, Ginger, and Parsley Juice:**

Ingredients: 4 or 5 carrots, 1/2 apple, 1 slice of ginger root (about 1/2 cm), and a handful of parsley.

Preparation: Cut the carrots and apples into pieces. Blend all the ingredients.

- **Potato, Carrot, Apple, and Parsley Juice:**

Ingredients: 1 slice of potato, 4 carrots, 1 apple, and a handful of parsley.

Preparation: Slice the potato into thin slices. Slice the carrots into strips 5 to 7 centimeters long. Slice the apple into thin slices, then blend all the ingredients.

- **Melon Smoothie:**

Ingredients: 2 slices of melon, with rind.

Preparation: Cut the melon into small pieces and blend. Consume 2 or 3 times a week on an empty stomach, half an hour or an hour before lunch.

- **Apple, Pear, and Sweet Turnip Juice:**

Ingredients: 1 apple, 1 pear, and 1 slice of sweet turnip (2.5 cm) (jicama).

Preparation: Cut the jicama into strips and the pear and apple into thin slices. Blend all the ingredients.

- **Carrot, Parsley, Celery, and Garlic Juice:**

Ingredients: 4 or 5 carrots, 1 bunch of parsley, 2 celery stalks, and 1 garlic clove.

Preparation: Compress the parsley and blend it with the rest of the ingredients, starting and ending with the carrots. Consume twice a day.

- **Grapefruit and Pineapple Juice:**

Ingredients: 1 grapefruit and 200 grams of peeled tropical pineapple.

Preparation: Peel the grapefruit, remove the white pith and seeds, and cut it into pieces. Cut the pineapple into pieces and blend everything.

- **Pineapple, Apple, and Ginger Juice:**

Ingredients: 1/4 pineapple with rind, 1/2 seedless apple, and 1 slice of ginger root (approximately 1/2 cm).

Preparation: Blend all the ingredients. Drink once a day.

- **Carrot, Apple, Celery, and Sweet Turnip Juice:**

Ingredients: 4 carrots, 1 apple, 1 celery stalk, and a 2.5 cm slice of sweet turnip (jicama).

Preparation: Clean the carrots and cut them into pieces 5 to 7 cm long. Cut the celery in the same manner. Slice the jicama into strips and the apple into thin slices. Blend all the ingredients.

- **Cherry, Lime, and Grape Juice:**

Ingredients: 1 bowl of pitted cherries, 1/4 bowl of lime, and a medium bunch of white grapes.

Preparation: Blend the cherries, grapes, and lime. Pour the juice into a glass and drink it once a day.

- **Kiwi, Lemon, Grape, and Celery Juice:**

Ingredients: 1 kiwi, 1/2 lemon, 100 grams of grapes, and 2 celery stalks.

Preparation: Peel and chop the kiwi. Peel the lemon, remove the white pith, cut it into quarters, and remove the seeds. Chop the celery. Blend all the ingredients.

- **Cabbage, Parsley, and Carrot Juice:**

Ingredients: 3 collard greens (or cabbage leaves), 1 bunch of parsley, and 4 or 5 carrots.

Preparation: Compress the cabbage leaves and parsley and blend them with the carrots. Consume 2 or 3 times a day.

- **Orange, Mango, and Cranberry Juice:**

Ingredients: 1/2 mango, 1/2 orange, 60 grams of cranberries, 1 teaspoon of honey, and 100 ml of water.

Preparation: Peel and dice the mango. Peel the orange, remove the white pith, and separate the segments. Blend all the ingredients. Add the water to the mixture.

- **Cherry Juice:**

Ingredients: 30 grams of cherries and 1 glass of water.

Preparation: Wash the cherries thoroughly, remove the stems, cut them in half, and remove the pits. Blend the cherries with the water.

MEDICINAL PLANTS

"Health is the best gift one can receive, and the one people pursue the least"
(Unknown author)

Since time immemorial, humanity has turned to the natural world for answers to its needs. Medicinal herbs, faithful companions on this journey, have generously shared their wisdom to ease ailments and enhance well-being. This ancient knowledge, carefully preserved through the ages, has found a renewed place in the modern world, offering a healthy and sustainable option to address today's challenges.

In a society increasingly conscious of the adverse effects of certain pharmaceutical treatments and the environmental toll of unsustainable practices, botanical remedies are experiencing a resurgence with renewed prominence. For those seeking a balanced, respectful lifestyle in harmony with the environment, these green treasures provide invaluable solutions. This revival not only reflects a growing interest in ecological approaches but also an evolution toward holistic care for both the body and the planet.

What makes these natural wonders truly extraordinary is the complexity of their compounds, capable of delivering antioxidant, anti-inflammatory, antibacterial, and antiviral properties, among others. Their potential ranges from alleviating everyday issues like sleeplessness or sluggish digestion to addressing conditions such as chronic stress or age-related ailments.

Beyond the ability to target specific concerns, these species serve as vital sources of micronutrients–vitamins, minerals, fiber, and antioxidants–that fortify the immune system and support long-term health. Incorporating them into dietary or self-care routines offers a simple, sustainable, and effective path toward illness prevention and enhanced overall wellness.

The botanical kingdom boasts remarkable diversity, featuring countless species uniquely suited to meet specific needs. Whether prepared as herbal teas, applied as balms or tinctures, or utilized in the form of essential oils, their applications are as versatile as they are effective, seamlessly fitting into various lifestyles.

More than mere remedies, these natural allies inspire us to reconnect with the world around us. Harnessing their benefits requires respect for environmental rhythms and a deeper appreciation for our planet's ecosystems. Each herb or extract serves as a tangible reminder of our connection to the living world, fostering a sense of harmony that transcends the physical and nurtures the spiritual.

In addition to their myriad health benefits, plant-based solutions stand out for their accessibility and practical versatility. Many species grow abundantly in wild habitats or can be easily cultivated in home gardens, offering an affordable, sustainable alternative. In a global context marked by economic inequalities, these wellness allies provide inclusive options to complement–or even replace–costly interventions.

Over the centuries, knowledge of these natural solutions has been carefully preserved through oral traditions and written records. This heritage, rooted in deep respect for biodiversity, has been bolstered by modern science, validating the effects of their active compounds and shedding light on their mechanisms of action. It represents a powerful synergy between tradition and innovation, broadening the therapeutic applications of these botanical marvels.

However, unlocking their full potential requires responsible use. Every human body is unique, and while these species possess well-documented therapeutic properties, they are not without risks. Misuse or interactions with conventional medications can lead to adverse effects. Therefore, obtaining accurate and reliable information is essential to ensure safe and effective usage.

One particularly fascinating aspect is how the components within a plant work in unison. Whole extracts, resulting from this intricate interaction, often produce more balanced and holistic effects compared to isolated compounds. Molecules interact in complementary ways, maximizing benefits while reducing potential side effects. Conversely, isolated active principles can provide concentrated solutions but may carry an increased risk of adverse effects on the body.

The innate harmony of these botanical wonders highlights one of biodiversity's greatest gifts—balance. Whole extracts are celebrated for their gentleness and ability to integrate seamlessly with the body's natural processes. On the other hand, synthesized compounds strive for potency, often at the expense of stability. The synergistic interaction between molecular components amplifies therapeutic benefits while limiting potential downsides, making them a choice deeply aligned with human needs.

Ultimately, medicinal plants transcend their role as therapeutic tools—they bridge ancestral wisdom and scientific innovation. They remind us that the health of our bodies and the well-being of our planet are profoundly interconnected. By safeguarding this invaluable legacy, we nurture not only our own health but also that of future generations, renewing the delicate balance between humanity and nature.

Essential Information

Although plants are natural in origin, they should not be considered entirely harmless. Their active compounds may cause adverse effects or trigger allergies in certain individuals.

Occasional consumption of an infusion is unlikely to cause harm. However, excessive, prolonged, or frequent use may result in discomfort, allergic reactions, or even toxicity.

Tolerance to natural remedies varies greatly among

individuals. If you are pregnant, breastfeeding, or managing conditions such as chronic illnesses, allergies, kidney or liver insufficiency, cancer, or undergoing medical treatment, it is crucial to refer to the section titled **"Learn Everything You Need to Know About the Plants"** before using them. This section provides essential information on potential risks, contraindications, and interactions, enabling you to make informed and responsible decisions.

Guidelines for Care with Herbal Remedies

For best results, continue using the remedies until your symptoms have completely disappeared. The treatment duration will vary depending on factors like the severity of your condition, how it progresses, your personal commitment, and other important influences.

Keep in mind that some plants or herbal remedies are not suited for continuous or long-term use. In such cases, you will always find specific instructions that address this.

While following the guidelines for the remedies below, it is just as important to focus on the underlying causes of your symptoms. To better understand the root of your health concerns, I recommend referring to the first chapter of this book, specifically the section titled "Causes," where you'll discover essential insights into tackling the problem at its source.

Finally, remember that patience is vital. A condition that has lingered for months or years cannot be resolved in just a few days. Stay committed, persevere, and always prioritize your health and well-being.

Measurements

To achieve the best results when preparing infusions, decoctions, or other plant-based recipes, it is essential to follow these dosage guidelines:

- A tablespoon refers to a level tablespoon.

• A teaspoon refers to a level teaspoon.

Effective Plants for External Use

It is crucial to note that if you have severe heart conditions, significant circulation issues, thrombophlebitis, or ulcers, you must consult your doctor before using any topical herbal remedies. Doing so will ensure that the treatment is both safe and suitable for your specific needs.

Additionally, please consider the following important precautions: **if you have open wounds, ulcers, inflamed and painful varicose veins, or blood clots in your legs, avoid massaging or applying pressure to the affected area.** Such actions could exacerbate your symptoms or further complicate your condition.

Below are some natural topical remedies designed to help relieve the discomfort associated with varicose veins:

• **Aloe Vera**: This plant is renowned for its soothing and refreshing properties, which help alleviate the pressure caused by varicose veins. Apply pure aloe vera gel and gently massage your legs in upward circular motions, starting at the ankles and working toward the knees.

• **Mint, Bay Leaf, and Chamomile**: Boil 2 liters of water and add a handful of mint leaves, bay leaves, and chamomile flowers. Allow the mixture to steep for 5 to 8 minutes. Once it has cooled to a comfortable temperature, pour it into a large container. Add a tablespoon of baking soda and soak your legs for at least 15 minutes. During this relaxing soak, you can gently massage your legs in upward movements to encourage better circulation.

• **Lavender Essential Oil**: Dilute a few drops of lavender essential oil in a carrier oil, such as almond or coconut oil. Gently massage your legs with the mixture. Lavender not only helps to relax tense muscles but also provides a refreshing and soothing sensation, enhancing your overall sense of well-being.

• **Ginger**: Prepare a concentrated infusion by boiling fresh slices of ginger in water for a few minutes. Allow the infusion to cool to a warm, comfortable temperature. Soak a clean cloth in the liquid, wring it out, and gently apply it to the affected areas. Ginger helps improve blood circulation and reduce inflammation, which can alleviate discomfort associated with varicose veins.

These remedies can complement your daily routine by promoting relaxation and providing relief from varicose vein discomfort. However, always consult with your healthcare provider before trying new treatments, especially if you have underlying health conditions.

Effective Plants for Internal Use

When it comes to relieving symptoms associated with varicose veins, nature provides a wide range of plants that have been shown to be highly effective. Below is a thoughtfully curated list of standout herbal options, organized alphabetically: **Butcher's broom, ginkgo biloba, horse chestnut, horsetail, red vine, and witch hazel.**

The best way to consume these plants is through infusions or decoctions, allowing you to harness their properties in the most natural way possible. If you prefer to sweeten these beverages, be sure to use only 100% natural stevia. Avoid other sweeteners that could alter their pure flavor or diminish their effectiveness.

Consistency is vital when assessing the effects of these plants. Select one option and use it for the suggested duration, or for at least three consecutive weeks, to evaluate its impact on your body. If you don't see significant improvements after this period, move on to another option from the list until you find the one that works best for you. Keep in mind that each individual is different and may respond uniquely to herbal treatments.

Below, you'll find a detailed description of each plant to help you understand its specific benefits. Scientific names (provided in parentheses) are included to avoid confusion, as many plants go by different common names depending on the region or country where they are grown. This ensures that you can identify the correct plant with confidence. Discover how these amazing plants can naturally enhance your health and well-being!

Butcher's broom (Ruscus aculeatus)

Decoction (of the root): Ingredients: 35 grams of root per liter of water. Place the root in the water and let it boil for 10 minutes. Drink it warm and unsweetened or with stevia. Drink 3 cups a day between meals.

Take this decoction for a maximum of 8 weeks, then rest for 4 weeks.

You can also consume it in the form of liquid extract, capsules, or tablets. The recommended dose is usually 300 to 600 mg per day, divided into two or three doses, but follow the manufacturer's instructions.

Ginkgo biloba (Ginkgo biloba L.)

Infusion: Ingredients: 50 grams of dried leaves in 500 ml of water. Boil the water, add the ginkgo, and let it steep for 8 minutes. Sweeten with honey or stevia. Drink 3 cups a day between meals.

Take this infusion for a maximum of 8 weeks, then rest for 4 weeks.

Ginkgo biloba can be found in the form of liquid extract, capsules, or tablets. In these cases, the recommended dose is usually 120 to 240 mg daily, divided into two doses. Follow the directions on the package.

Horse Chestnut (Aesculus hippocastanum)

Decoction: The ingredients are 30 grams (2 tablespoons) of dried horse chestnut bark and 1 liter of water. Preparation: Heat the water and add the horse chestnut when it begins to boil. Let it cook for 10 minutes. Remove from heat and consume when lukewarm. If possible, consume it unsweetened or with stevia. Divide into 2 or 3 servings per day after meals.

It would be best to take this decoction for a maximum of four weeks and then rest for another three weeks. During this break, you can try another of the plants recommended in this book.

You can also consume horse chestnut in the form of liquid extract, capsules, or tablets. In these cases, the recommended dose is usually 300 to 600 mg per day, divided into two or three doses, but follow the directions on the package.

Horsetail (Equisetum arvense)

Decoction: Ingredients: 4 tablespoons of dried plant in a liter and a half of water. Preparation: Cook over low heat for 30 minutes. Let cool, strain, and drink a cup in the morning and another at noon, away from meals.

Infusion: Add 2 tablespoons of horsetail per cup of boiling water and let it steep for 5 minutes. Drink 2 to 3 cups a day, away from meals.

It would be best to take this infusion for a maximum of four weeks and then rest for another eight weeks. During this break, you can try another of the plants recommended in this book.

Remarks: Avoid taking horsetail after 6 p.m. Because it is a diuretic, it may cause you to wake up during the night with the urge to urinate. Since diuresis can cause potassium loss, if you intend to continue taking horsetail for a prolonged period, you should supplement the treatment with potassium tablets.

Red vine (Vitis vinifera)

Decoction No. 1: Ingredients: 3 tablespoons of shredded dried leaves per liter of water. Preparation: Place the leaves in the water and bring to a boil. Let it boil for 15 minutes. Drink 2 or 3 glasses a day between meals.

Decoction No. 2 (for acute crises of pain or heaviness):

Ingredients: 1 teaspoon of dried leaves per cup of water. Preparation: Place the leaves in the water and boil them for 10 minutes. Remove from heat and let stand for 10 more minutes. Take 1 tablespoon every 15 minutes (to reduce varicose veins).

Take these for a maximum of 8 weeks and then rest for 4 weeks.

Witch hazel (Hamamelis virginiana)

Infusion: Ingredients: 1 teaspoon of dried witch hazel per cup of water. Heat the water, and when it boils, turn off the heat and add the witch hazel. Cover and let it steep for 10 to 15 minutes–drink unsweetened or with stevia. Drink 2 cups a day between meals.

Take this infusion for a maximum of 8 weeks, then rest for 4 weeks.

Herbal Remedy Recipes

Although the plants mentioned above are effective when used individually, their properties can be further enhanced when combined properly. Below are some particularly effective combinations.

- **Herbal Remedy Recipe No. 1**

Ingredients: Witch hazel, ginkgo biloba, horse chestnut, and butcher's broom. Use the four plants in equal parts.

Preparation: Use two teaspoons of this dried herb mixture per 500 ml of water. Add the plants and bring the water to a boil. Boil for 3 minutes. Remove the plants and let the mixture steep for an additional 15 minutes. Drink the mixture throughout the day, between meals.

- **Herbal Remedy Recipe No. 2**

Ingredients: 1 liter of water, 5 tablespoons of horsetail, 2 tablespoons of ginger root, 3 tablespoons of horse chestnut, and 1 teaspoon of mallow (leaves and flowers).

Preparation: Chop the ginger into thin slices and bring the water to a boil. Boil for 8 minutes, then remove from the heat. Add the other three plants, cover, and let steep for 15 minutes. Take three times a day, 30 minutes before meals.

- **Herbal Remedy Recipe No. 3**

Ingredients: Ginkgo biloba, butcher's broom, horsetail, and horse chestnut. Use 3 tablespoons of dried horsetail, 2 tablespoons of ginkgo biloba, 2 tablespoons of butcher's broom, and 2 tablespoons of horse chestnut.

Preparation: Combine the dried plants in equal parts. Use 2 teaspoons of the mixture per 500 ml of water. Bring the water to a boil, add the herbal mixture, and boil gently for 5 minutes. Remove from heat, cover, and let it steep for 10 minutes. Strain the infusion and drink 2 cups per day–one in the morning and one in the evening.

- **Herbal Remedy Recipe No. 4**

Ingredients: Witch hazel, red vine leaves, and butcher's broom. Use 4 tablespoons of red vine leaves, 3 tablespoons of witch hazel, and 2 tablespoons of butcher's broom.

Preparation: Mix all the dried herbs together. Use 3 teaspoons of this blend per 1 liter of boiling water. Once the water is boiling, pour it over the herbal blend, cover, and let it steep for 15 minutes. Strain the liquid and consume throughout the day in small quantities, preferably between meals, for better absorption.

Note: At the end of this chapter, you will find a detailed explanation of the potential effects of all the plants mentioned. Be sure to review this section carefully before consuming any of them.

Simple Steps to Make a Tincture for Varicose Veins

Tinctures, also known as concentrated botanical extracts, provide an effective and powerful way to harness the therapeutic benefits of medicinal plants. Through a meticulous extraction process, essential compounds–such as phytochemicals and active principles–are captured, concentrating their valuable healing properties.

For centuries, these liquid solutions have been a cornerstone of traditional medicine, prized for their proven efficacy and remarkable versatility. In recent years, they have regained widespread popularity, driven by the growing interest in natural remedies and herbal practices.

The process of preparing tinctures can vary, but it generally involves immersing specific plant parts–such as roots, leaves, flowers, or bark–in a solvent like alcohol, glycerin, or water. During this steeping phase, the plant's active components are extracted and infused into the liquid, transforming it into a medicinal concentrate that preserves its vital properties.

One of the most notable advantages of tinctures is their practicality. They are incredibly easy to use: just add a few drops to water or juice for quick, effective absorption. Their high concentration also allows for precise dosing, making it simple to tailor usage to individual needs.

- **Making a Butcher's Broom Tincture:**
Ingredients:
   - 40 grams of butcher's broom root
   - 200 ml of vodka or brandy (apple cider vinegar or vegetable glycerin can be used instead for those who cannot consume alcohol)
   - A glass bottle of approximately 200 ml with an airtight cap
   - A dark brown dropper bottle to protect it from light

Preparation:
1. Peel the butcher's broom and slice or grate it. Place it in the airtight glass jar, filling about half of the jar.
2. Add the vodka, brandy, or vinegar to the jar, filling it. Shake well to ensure a good mixture.
3. Store the jar in a dark, warm place away from heat sources. Let the mixture macerate for at least 3 weeks, although it can also be left to macerate for several months. Be sure to shake the

jar once a week and put it away again.

4. After the maceration period, filter the tincture using sterilized cotton gauze into a glass container.

5. Transfer the filtered tincture to the brown glass dropper bottle and seal tightly. Label the bottle with the date of bottling.

Dosage: The recommended dose for adults is 30 drops, 3 times a day, for a maximum of 4 consecutive weeks. After this period, a 1-month break is recommended before resuming treatment, which consists of 4 weeks of treatment followed by a 1-month break.

Storage: Keep the tincture in a cool, dark place, and make sure to check the expiration date (1 year).

Learn Everything You Need to Know About the Plants

In this section, we'll delve into the most recommended botanical species for treating the condition at hand. You'll find essential information about their possible adverse effects, contraindications, and interactions, as well as detailed insights into each plant. From their descriptions and habitats to their uses, chemical components, histories, and therapeutic properties, this chapter is designed to take you on a fascinating journey of discovery.

My goal is to provide you with a comprehensive understanding of these plants, helping you grasp their context and fully appreciate their many benefits. We'll explore their historical origins and significance in traditional medicine, highlighting their invaluable role in natural care.

I want you to become an expert on these species, capable of making informed decisions in your pursuit of wellness. Get ready to expand your knowledge and uncover the extraordinary healing power of nature!

Butcher's broom (Ruscus aculeatus)

Description:
Butcher's broom, scientifically known as Ruscus aculeatus, is a perennial plant belonging to the Liliaceae family. It is native to Europe and parts of Asia and is characterized as a shrub with stiff evergreen leaves. Its stems are green and branched, with needle-like spines on its leaves, which have earned it the common name of butcher's broom. It produces small greenish flowers and red fruits in the form of berries.

Habitat and cultivation:
Butcher's broom is found mainly in wooded and shady areas, where it can grow in moist, well-drained soils. It is commonly found in oak, beech, and pine forests. It can be grown in gardens and containers, preferring acidic soils and partial or complete shade.

Parts used:
The roots and rhizomes are mainly used for medicinal purposes. These parts of the plant contain various beneficial compounds that have therapeutic properties.

Components:
It contains several active components, including steroids, saponins, flavonoids, and tannins. These compounds are responsible for the plant's medicinal properties.

History and tradition:
Traditional European medicine has long used it. Since ancient times, it has been valued for its diuretic, anti-inflammatory, and vagotonic properties. Additionally, it has been used to treat circulatory problems, such as venous insufficiency and hemorrhoids.

Therapeutic properties:
Phytotherapy uses it due to its therapeutic properties. It is attributed to benefits such as improving blood circulation, strengthening veins and capillaries, reducing inflammation, and relieving symptoms of hemorrhoids. It has also been used to treat lymphatic system disorders and alleviate tired legs and varicose veins symptoms.

Curiosities:
Butcher's broom has some interesting curiosities associated with it. For example, although it is called a butcher's broom because of the thorns on its leaves, it does not belong to the family of hot plants like chili peppers. Additionally, the red berries of butcher's broom are poisonous to humans, so they should not be consumed.

Adverse or side effects:
Although butcher's broom is generally safe when used properly, some mild adverse effects have been reported in isolated cases. These may include stomach upset, nausea, diarrhea, or allergic reactions in sensitive individuals. If any side effects are experienced, use should be discontinued.

Contraindications:
Although it is considered safe for most people, there are some contraindications. Its use is not recommended for pregnant or breastfeeding women due to the lack of sufficient evidence on its safety during these stages. Additionally, people with kidney or heart disorders, as well as those taking anticoagulant medications, should avoid using butcher's broom without consulting a physician.

Interactions:
Butcher's broom may interact with certain medications and herbs, so caution is essential when combining it with other treatments. It may potentiate the effects of anticoagulant drugs, such as warfarin, increasing the risk of bleeding. Additionally, it may interfere with iron absorption, so it is recommended to separate the intake of iron supplements from the intake of butcher's broom.

Ginger (Zingiber officinale)

Description:
Ginger is a perennial plant with underground stems called rhizomes. It has long, narrow leaves and yellow or white cone-shaped flowers. The rhizome is the most commonly used part

and has a spicy and aromatic flavor.

Habitat and cultivation:

Ginger is native to tropical Asia and is grown in many parts of the world. It prefers warm, humid climates and can be cultivated both in gardens and in pots indoors.

Parts used:

The rhizome of ginger is the most commonly used part. It is harvested, peeled, and used fresh or dried for culinary and medicinal purposes. The leaves and flowers can also be used in specific preparations.

Components:

It contains active compounds such as gingerol, shogaol, and zingiberene, which give it its medicinal properties. It also contains antioxidants, vitamins, and minerals.

Ginger, scientifically known as Zingiber officinale, is a perennial plant native to tropical Asia. Due to its numerous health benefits, it has been used for centuries as a spice in cooking and traditional medicine.

History and tradition:

This plant has been cultivated and used in Asia for over 5,000 years. It is believed to have originated in the coastal region of South Asia, specifically in what is today India and China. From there, it spread to various parts of the world and integrated into many cultures' culinary and medicinal traditions.

Ginger is especially valued in traditional Asian medicine, such as Ayurvedic and Chinese medicine. In these traditions, it is considered a "hot" plant that can help balance the body and treat various ailments. It has been used to relieve digestive problems, such as nausea, vomiting, and upset stomach. Additionally, it has been used as a general tonic to strengthen the immune system and promote blood circulation.

Therapeutic properties:

It contains bioactive compounds, such as gingerols and

shogaols, which give it its medicinal properties. These compounds are responsible for ginger's characteristic flavor and aroma and benefit the human body.

One of ginger's most well-known properties is its ability to relieve nausea and vomiting. Numerous studies have shown that ginger consumption can be effective in relieving nausea caused by pregnancy, chemotherapy, or surgery. The compounds in ginger act on the digestive system, reducing discomfort and improving intestinal motility.

Additionally, ginger has been used to relieve pain and inflammation. Gingerols and shogaols have been shown to have anti-inflammatory and analgesic properties, making them a natural choice for pain relief in conditions such as arthritis, muscle aches, and migraines. Some studies even suggest that regular consumption of ginger may help reduce chronic inflammation in the body.

Ginger may also have positive effects on cardiovascular health. Regular consumption of ginger has been suggested to help reduce cholesterol and triglyceride levels in the blood and improve blood circulation. These effects could contribute to heart health and reduce the risk of cardiovascular disease.

In addition to its therapeutic properties, ginger is also used as a spice in cooking due to its spicy and aromatic flavor. It is added to savory and sweet dishes, as well as to beverages such as ginger tea. Its culinary versatility makes it popular in many cultures and cuisines worldwide.

Curiosities:
Ginger is a plant native to tropical Asia. It has been used for centuries both in cooking and traditional medicine due to its medicinal properties. Here are some interesting facts:

Spicy and refreshing flavor: Ginger has a distinctive taste with a spicy and refreshing touch. This characteristic flavor is due to active compounds such as gingerols and shogaols, which also give it its medicinal properties.

Ancient use: Ginger has been used in traditional Chinese and Indian medicine for over 2,000 years. It has been employed to treat a wide variety of conditions, from digestive problems to muscle aches and colds.

Culinary use: Besides its medicinal properties, ginger is a popular cooking spice. It is used in sweet and savory dishes, such as curries, desserts, infusions, and refreshing drinks like ginger ale.

Adverse or side effects:

Although ginger is generally safe for most people when consumed in moderate amounts, some individuals may experience adverse side effects:

Upset stomach: Excessive consumption of ginger may cause an upset stomach, nausea, heartburn, or diarrhea in some people. These side effects are usually mild and resolve on their own.

Interference with medications: Ginger may interact with certain medications, such as anticoagulants or antihypertensives. Caution is advised when combining ginger with these medications; it is vital to consult a physician beforehand.

Allergic reactions: Although rare, some people may be allergic to ginger. This can manifest as skin rashes, itching, swelling, or difficulty breathing. If any allergic reaction occurs, seek medical attention immediately.

Contraindications:

There are contraindications to consider when using ginger:

Coagulation disorders: Because ginger inhibits platelet aggregation, caution should be exercised when consuming it in people with coagulation disorders or those taking anticoagulant drugs. A physician should be consulted before use.

Pregnancy and lactation: Although it has been traditionally used to treat morning sickness, caution is advised during pregnancy and lactation. A physician should be consulted before using ginger during these stages.

Interactions:
It can interact with certain medications and supplements, so it is essential to use caution when combining it with other treatments. Some known interactions include:

Anticoagulants: Ginger, due to its ability to inhibit platelet aggregation, may increase the risk of bleeding when combined with anticoagulant medications such as warfarin. Medical supervision is recommended if both treatments are used.

Antihypertensives: Ginger may have hypotensive effects, which could interact with high blood pressure medications. If you are taking medicines for hypertension, exercise caution and consult a physician before using ginger.

Ginkgo biloba

Description:
Ginkgo biloba is an ancient tree that has existed for millions of years. It is considered a living fossil because of its unique appearance, which includes fan-shaped leaves and spreading branches. The tree can reach a height of up to 30 meters and has smooth, grayish bark. Its leaves are bright green in summer and turn golden in autumn before falling.

Habitat and cultivation:
Ginkgo biloba originated in China and has been cultivated in Asia for centuries. Today, it is found in many parts of the world, including Europe and North America. It prefers temperate climates and adapts well to different soil types. It is a hardy tree that can grow in urban and rural areas.

Parts used:
In medicinal terms, the parts of Ginkgo biloba primarily used are the leaves and seeds. The leaves are harvested in autumn and dried for later use. However, the seeds are used to a lesser extent and must be processed appropriately, as they contain

raw toxic substances.

Components:
Ginkgo biloba contains a variety of active constituents, the most notable being flavonoids and terpenoids. Flavonoids are known for their antioxidant properties, while terpenoids, such as ginkgolides and bilobalides, have neuroprotective effects and improve blood circulation.

History and tradition:
Ginkgo biloba has a rich history and a long tradition in Chinese medicine. It has been used for centuries to treat various conditions, such as memory problems, respiratory issues, and circulatory disorders. Additionally, the Ginkgo tree is considered sacred in some cultures, and spiritual and longevity properties are attributed to it.

Therapeutic properties:
Ginkgo biloba has been widely studied for its therapeutic properties. It improves blood circulation and oxygen flow to the brain, which may benefit memory and cognitive function. It has also been used to treat vision problems, tinnitus (ringing in the ears), and vertigo. However, it is essential to note that Ginkgo biloba supplements are not without side effects and may interact with certain medications.

Curiosities:
Ginkgo biloba is a fascinating species with several curiosities associated with it. For example, it is considered a "living fossil" because it has survived for millions of years without significant changes in its structure. Additionally, it is a highly resilient tree, capable of surviving pollution, diseases, and adverse weather conditions. It is also interesting to note that Ginkgo biloba leaves have a unique shape and are used in Chinese culture in the preparation of traditional dishes.

Adverse or side effects:
Although Ginkgo biloba is generally safe for most people when consumed in adequate doses, some adverse effects may occur in rare cases. These side effects may include headaches, stomach upset, dizziness, diarrhea, nausea, or allergic

reactions in some people. Additionally, due to its anticoagulant effect, there is a risk of excessive bleeding in people who are taking anticoagulants or have clotting disorders. Caution is advised in people with seizures, clotting disorders, or those undergoing surgery.

Contraindications:
Although it is widely used, some contraindications must be considered. It is not recommended for pregnant or lactating women due to the lack of evidence on its safety in these cases. Additionally, people with a known allergy to Ginkgo biloba or its components should avoid taking it. Caution should also be exercised in people with seizure disorders, coagulation disorders, or those scheduled for surgery soon, as Ginkgo may interact with drugs and increase the risk of complications.

Interactions:
Ginkgo may interact with certain medications, which may affect their effectiveness or increase the risk of adverse effects. For example, it may increase the risk of bleeding when taken with anticoagulants such as warfarin or aspirin. Additionally, it may interfere with the action of certain drugs used to treat seizure disorders, such as carbamazepine. It may also interact with drugs that affect liver function, such as some anti-depressants and HIV medications. Therefore, informing your doctor or pharmacist if you are taking Ginkgo biloba is essential to avoid possible harmful interactions.

Horse chestnut (Aesculus hippocastanum)

Description:
The horse chestnut is a medium-to-large tree that can reach heights up to 30 meters. It has a straight trunk and spreading branches that form a rounded crown. Its leaves are large, compound, and palmate in shape, with 5 to 7 leaflets with serrated edges. During the spring, the tree produces flowers in the form of erect white or pale pink spikes. The fruits of the horse chestnut are spiny capsules containing shiny, dark brown

seeds.

Habitat and Cultivation:
Horse chestnut is native to the Balkans and Asia Minor mountain regions but is now cultivated in many parts of the world. It prefers temperate to cool climates and well-drained soils. It is commonly found in parks, avenues, and gardens, and its wood is also used in furniture and planting.

Parts Used:
Regarding therapeutic use, the most commonly used parts of the horse chestnut are the seeds and the bark. The seeds are highly valued and are used in the preparation of extracts and tinctures. The bark can also be used as a decoction or tincture.

Components:
Horse chestnut seeds contain various compounds, among which triterpene saponosides, such as escin, stand out. Escin is considered the primary active component responsible for the therapeutic properties of horse chestnut. Flavonoids, tannins, and other bioactive compounds are also found in smaller quantities.

History and Tradition:
Horse chestnut has been used in herbal medicine for centuries. It is believed to have been introduced to Europe from Asia in the 16th century. Traditionally, it has been used to treat circulatory problems such as venous insufficiency, varicose veins, and capillary fragility. It has also been used topically to relieve inflammation and pain related to bruises, contusions, and hematomas.

Therapeutic Properties:
Horse chestnut is mainly used for its vagotonic and vasoprotective properties. The escin present in the seeds strengthens blood vessels, improves circulation, and reduces swelling. This makes it a popular natural remedy for treating venous disorders such as varicose veins, chronic venous insufficiency, and heavy legs.

In addition to its venotonic properties, horse chestnut may

also have antioxidant and anti-inflammatory effects.

Curiosities:
The horse chestnut is known by its scientific name, Aesculus hippocastanum, where "Aesculus" comes from Latin and refers to a type of oak tree, while "hippocastanum" means "horse chestnut". This name originates from the ancient tradition of feeding the tree's seeds to horses.

Despite its name, "horse chestnut" has no relation to the common chestnut. The name arose because it was brought to Europe from Asia by Portuguese colonizers and was mistakenly associated with the East Indies.

In some cultures, especially in Eastern Europe, horse chestnut seeds have historically been used to make amulets and talismans, which were believed to protect against the evil eye and other negative energies.

Adverse or Side Effects:
Although horse chestnut is generally well-tolerated, adverse effects may occur in some individuals. The most common include stomach upset, nausea, vomiting, and headache. These side effects are usually mild and resolve on their own.

In rare cases, allergic reactions have been reported. If you experience symptoms such as a rash, itching, swelling, or difficulty breathing after consumption, it is vital to seek medical attention immediately.

Contraindications:
Individuals with liver or kidney disease, as well as those with bleeding disorders or gastric ulcers, should avoid using horse chestnut, as it may worsen these conditions.

Due to its potential to affect blood coagulation, horse chestnuts should be used cautiously when taking anticoagulant or antiplatelet medications, such as warfarin. In these cases, it is essential to consult a physician before use.

Interactions:

Horse chestnut may interact with certain medications, such as anticoagulants, antiplatelet agents, and nonsteroidal anti-inflammatory drugs (NSAIDs). It may increase the risk of bleeding or interfere with the effectiveness of these medications. If you take any of them, you must talk to your doctor before using horse chestnut.

Additionally, horse chestnuts have been reported to interact with blood pressure medications, diuretics, and medications that affect liver function. Therefore, it is advisable to consult a healthcare professional before combining them.

Horsetail (Equisetum arvense)

Description:
Horsetail is a perennial plant belonging to the genus Equisetum. It is characterized by hollow, jointed stems that resemble horse tails. It has small leaves and cone-shaped spores at the top of the stems.

Habitat and Cultivation:
Horsetail is commonly found in wet and marshy areas worldwide. It grows in mineral-rich soils and can tolerate various light and water conditions. Horsetail can be cultivated in gardens and is also found in the wild.

Parts Used:
The parts of horsetail used are the sterile stems that grow in spring before the appearance of spores. These stems are harvested and used both fresh and dried for their medicinal properties.

Components:
Horsetail contains several beneficial components, such as silica, flavonoids, minerals (including potassium and calcium), ascorbic acid (vitamin C), and alkaloids. Silica is a primary component contributing to the plant's healing properties.

History and Tradition:
Horsetail has been used in traditional medicine for centuries due to its medicinal properties and health benefits. It is a perennial plant found in various parts of the world, including Europe, Asia, and North America. Its name comes from its appearance, as its stems resemble horse tails.

This plant has been valued in the history and traditions of different cultures. In ancient Rome, for example, it was believed to have healing properties and was used to treat wounds and urinary problems. It was also used to treat various ailments in traditional Chinese and Indian Ayurvedic medicine.

In addition to its medicinal uses, horsetail has also been used in agriculture and gardening due to its silica content, which strengthens plant tissues and promotes growth. It has also been used to reinforce fabric fibers in the manufacture of cosmetic products and in the textile industry.

Therapeutic Properties:
Horsetail is known for its therapeutic properties and health benefits. Some of its most notable properties are:

Natural Diuretic: Horsetail has a mild diuretic effect, stimulating urine production and helping to eliminate toxins and waste from the body. This can be beneficial in treating fluid retention, reducing swelling, and promoting kidney health.

Bone and Tissue Strengthening: Horsetail contains silica, a mineral in high concentrations in this plant. Silica is essential for the formation and strengthening of connective tissues, such as bones, cartilage, and nails. It can also help promote healthy skin, hair, and teeth.

Anti-inflammatory Properties: Horsetail has anti-inflammatory properties, which may help reduce inflammation in the body. This can be beneficial in treating inflammatory conditions, such as arthritis and inflammatory bowel disease.

Improving Urinary System Health: Horsetail has traditionally been used to treat urinary system conditions, such as urinary tract infections and kidney stones. Its diuretic effect can help cleanse and detoxify the kidneys, promoting kidney health and preventing stone formation.

Antioxidant Action: Horsetail contains antioxidants that help protect cells from damage caused by free radicals. Free radicals are unstable molecules that can damage DNA and contribute to aging and various diseases. The antioxidants present in horsetail help neutralize these free radicals and protect the body against oxidative stress.

Horsetail can be consumed as an infusion, in capsules, or as liquid extracts.

Curiosities:

Horsetail is a perennial herb that grows in wet, marshy areas worldwide. It gets its name from its distinctive appearance, resembling the bristles of a horse's tail. Besides its peculiar appearance, horsetail has several interesting curiosities:

Living Fossils: Horsetails are considered living fossils, as they are plants that have existed on Earth for millions of years. The first horsetail species is believed to have emerged more than 300 million years ago, during the Carboniferous period.

Silica Content: Horsetail is one of the few plants containing high levels of silica, an essential mineral component for human health. This makes it popular in traditional medicine for strengthening hair, nails, and bones.

Use in Gardening: Horsetail is also appreciated for its medicinal properties. Its hollow, jointed stems give it a unique structure, and it is often used as an ornamental plant in water gardens or to create natural borders in flower beds.

Adverse or Side Effects:

Despite its potential benefits, horsetail may have some adverse effects in some instances. Some of these include:

Thiaminase Toxicity: Horsetail contains an enzyme called thiaminase, which can interfere with the absorption of vitamin

B1 (thiamine). This can lead to thiamine deficiency if consumed in large amounts or for prolonged periods.

Interference with Medications: Horsetail may interact with certain medications, such as diuretics or blood thinners. If you take any medication, consult a physician before using the plant to avoid negative interactions.

Allergic Reactions: Some people may be allergic to horsetail. This allergy may manifest as rashes, itching, swelling, or difficulty breathing. If you experience any allergic reaction, seek immediate medical attention.

Contraindications:

There are contraindications to consider when using horsetail:

Pregnancy and Lactation: The safety of horsetail during pregnancy and lactation has not been sufficiently investigated. As a precaution, it is recommended that pregnant or nursing women avoid use or consult a physician before use.

Kidney Problems: Due to its silica content and diuretic capacity, horsetail may aggravate kidney problems, such as kidney stones or kidney failure. Therefore, caution is advised for people with kidney problems.

Interactions:

Horsetail can interact with certain medications, so it is essential to use caution when combining it with other treatments. Some known interactions include:

Diuretic Medications: Horsetail has natural diuretic pro-perties so that it could increase the diuretic effect of diuretic medications. This could lead to excessive fluid and mineral loss in the body.

Anticoagulants: Horsetail may have mild anticoagulant effects, which could increase the risk of bleeding when combined with anticoagulant medications such as warfarin. Medical supervision is recommended if both treatments are used.

Mallow (Malva sylvestris)

Description:
Mallow is a perennial herbaceous plant in the Malvaceae family. Its erect, branched stem can reach a height of up to 1 meter. Its leaves are large, palmate, and toothed, bright green. The funnel-shaped flowers vary in color from pale pink to deep purple. This plant is known for its beauty and is used in ornamental gardens and traditional medicine.

Habitat and Cultivation:
Mallow is native to Europe and is commonly found in meadows, roadsides, and wastelands. It adapts to different types of soils, although it prefers well-drained, nutrient-rich soils. This plant can grow in temperate and warm climates, tolerating both direct sunlight and partial shade. Mallow is easily propagated by seed and can also be grown from cuttings.

Parts Used:
Mallow leaves and flowers are mainly used for medicinal purposes. The leaves are harvested when the plant is fully grown, while the flowers are harvested when fully open. The dried parts of the plant are then used to prepare infusions, extracts, or ointments.

Components:
Mallow contains several bioactive components that give it its therapeutic properties. These include mucilages, which are gel-like substances with emollient and softening properties. It also contains flavonoids, antioxidants, and phenolic compounds, which may have anti-inflammatory and antioxidant effects.

History and Tradition:
Mallow has been used in traditional medicine for centuries. Ancient Egyptians and Greeks, for example, are believed to have used it to treat respiratory diseases, skin irritations, and digestive problems. Additionally, some traditions consider it a sacred plant and attribute it with protective and magical

properties.

Therapeutic Properties:
Mallow is used in herbal medicine due to its therapeutic properties. It is attributed with anti-inflammatory, emollient, soothing, and healing properties. Therefore, it is used to treat respiratory conditions such as coughs and colds, as well as digestive problems like gastritis and heartburn. It is also used topically to relieve skin irritation, such as minor burns, rashes, and insect bites.

Curiosities:
Mallow, also known as Malva sylvestris, is a herbaceous perennial plant with some interesting curiosities associated with it. For example, mallow has been used since ancient times for its medicinal properties and was attributed with magical and protective qualities. Additionally, this plant is known for its beauty, as it produces showy flowers in shades ranging from light pink to deep purple.

Adverse or Side Effects:
Although mallow is generally considered safe, adverse or side effects may occur in rare cases. Some people may experience allergic reactions when coming in contact with the plant or consuming its parts. Additionally, excessive consumption of mallow may have a laxative effect and cause diarrhea. It is important to note that, as with any medicinal plant, it is advisable to use it in moderation and consult a health professional if adverse effects occur.

Contraindications:
There are no significant contraindications, but caution is advised in some instances. For example, people with a history of allergies or sensitivity to other plants of the Malvaceae family may be at increased risk of developing allergic reactions to mallow. Additionally, it is advised to avoid the use of mallow during pregnancy and lactation, as there have not been enough studies to determine its safety during these stages.

Interactions:
Mallow has not been associated with significant drug or

supplement interactions. However, it is always advisable to consult a healthcare professional if you are taking any medications or have pre-existing health conditions before using Mallow therapeutically. This is especially relevant if you take anticoagulants or medicines that may interact with herbs or medicinal plants.

Red vine (Vitis vinifera)

Red vine is a climbing plant in the Vitaceae family. It is known for its deep red grapes and its use in wine production.

Description:
Red vine is a perennial plant that can grow to considerable heights, reaching over 10 meters in length under favorable conditions. Its leaves are large, lobed, and have serrated edges. The leaves turn red in autumn, giving them their common name. The clusters of grapes produced by the red vine are small and contain round or ellipsoidal dark red or purple berries.

Habitat and cultivation:
Red vine is native to the Mediterranean region but is now cultivated in many parts of the world. It requires a temperate climate and well-drained soils to grow appropriately. The vine is mainly grown for its grapes, which are used in wine production but can also be consumed fresh.

Parts used:
The leaves and grapes are the most commonly used parts of red vine for therapeutic purposes. The leaves are harvested during the summer and dried for later use in infusions and extracts, while the grapes can also be used to prepare home remedies.

Components:
It leaves contain several bioactive compounds, including flavonoids like quercetin and rutin. These compounds are known for their antioxidant and anti-inflammatory properties.

Tannins, organic acids, and minerals such as potassium and calcium are also found in the leaves.

History and tradition:
Humans have cultivated and used the red vine for thousands of years. Its cultivation dates back to ancient Mesopotamia and Egypt, where it was valued for its grapes and for its symbolic and ceremonial significance. Throughout history, the red vine has been associated with celebration, good health, and longevity.

Therapeutic properties:
Due to its therapeutic properties, it has traditionally been used in herbal medicine. It is considered helpful in improving blood circulation, strengthening capillary vessels, and reducing capillary fragility and permeability. It is also attributed with antioxidant and anti-inflammatory properties, which may contribute to cardiovascular health and alleviate symptoms of circulatory disorders such as varicose veins and venous insufficiency.

Curiosities:
Red vine is one of the oldest plants cultivated by humans, with cultivation estimated to date back more than 6,000 years.

Red vine grapes are used in wine production, juices, herbal medicine, jams, and other gastronomic products.

Red vine is a vigorous climbing plant and can cover large areas, forming dense vines in vineyards.

Adverse or side effects:
Although red vine is generally considered safe for most people, mild adverse effects, such as stomach upset, nausea, or diarrhea, may occur in some cases. These side effects are uncommon and usually temporary.

Some people may have allergic reactions to red vine. If you experience symptoms such as itching, swelling, or difficulty breathing after consumption, seek medical attention immediately.

Contraindications:
Red vine may have anticoagulant and antiplatelet effects, which means it can interfere with blood clotting. Therefore, people taking anticoagulant or antiplatelet medications, such as warfarin, should avoid excessive consumption of red vine or consult their physician before doing so.

Due to a lack of sufficient information, red vine should be used cautiously during pregnancy and lactation. Before using it during these stages, consult a health professional.

Interactions:
Red Vine may interact with certain medications, such as anticoagulants, antiplatelet drugs, nonsteroidal anti-inflammatory drugs (NSAIDs), and blood pressure medications. It may potentiate the effects of these medications, which may increase the risk of bleeding or affect the effectiveness of blood pressure medications. If you are taking any of these medications, it is essential to talk to your doctor before consuming red vine.

Witch hazel (Hamamelis virginiana)

Description:
Witch hazel, scientifically known as Hamamelis virginiana, is a shrub or small tree native to North America. It is characterized by its showy flowers and colorful foliage in autumn. Witch hazel has alternate, simple, toothed leaves, and its flowers are bright yellow or orange. It is known for its ability to bloom in winter and early spring, making it a popular ornamental plant.

Habitat and Cultivation:
Witch hazel is found naturally in moist forests and swamps in North America, mainly in the eastern and central regions of the United States. It prefers humus-rich, well-drained soils. For cultivation, it can be planted in gardens and parks, as long as it is provided with a suitable environment with partial shade and moist soil. It is a hardy plant and can tolerate cold weather.

Parts Used:
In medicinal terms, witch hazel's main parts are the leaves and bark. The leaves are harvested in autumn and dried for later use. On the other hand, the bark is obtained from young branches and dried for use. These parts contain active compounds with therapeutic properties.

Components:
Witch hazel contains various beneficial components, including tannins, flavonoids, and volatile oils. Tannins are astringent and help reduce inflammation and skin irritation. Flavonoids possess antioxidant and anti-inflammatory properties, and volatile oils give the plant a distinctive aroma.

History and Tradition:
Witch hazel has a long history of use in traditional medicine. Native Americans, such as the Iroquois and Mohicans, used it to treat a variety of conditions, including skin problems, hemorrhoids, and muscle pain. It was also used in rituals and ceremonies. Today, witch hazel has become popular as an ingredient in skincare products and is used in topical treatments to soothe irritation and promote healing.

Therapeutic Properties:
Witch hazel has long been used for its therapeutic properties. It is credited with astringent, anti-inflammatory, and hemostatic actions. It is commonly used to relieve skin discomforts such as insect bites, sunburn, rashes, and irritated skin. Due to its properties in reducing inflammation and relieving pain, witch hazel is also used to treat hemorrhoids. Additionally, it can help stimulate blood circulation and promote the healing of minor wounds.

Curiosities:
Witch hazel is associated with some exciting curiosities. For example, it is known as the "witches' tree" because of its ability to bloom in the dead of winter, which was considered a magical power in ancient times. Its flowers have a unique shape, with slender, ribbon-like petals that curve back, giving them a distinctive appearance. It is also interesting to note that witch hazel is used in the cosmetic industry and is found in a variety

of skin care products due to its beneficial properties.

Adverse or Side Effects:
Although it is generally safe for most people when used topically, some adverse effects may occur in rare cases. These side effects include skin irritation, redness, itching, or allergic reactions in some sensitive individuals. To check for adverse reactions, it is essential to perform a patch test on a small skin area before using products containing witch hazel.

Contraindications:
Although it is considered safe for topical use, there are some contraindications to be aware of. It is not recommended for use in people with known allergies to witch hazel or any of its components. Also, topical use on open wounds or damaged skin should be avoided as it may cause additional irritation. It is best to consult a healthcare professional if you are pregnant or nursing.

Interactions:
In general, witch hazel has no significant interactions with medications or other herbs. However, it is essential to use caution when using witch hazel products with other topical products to avoid possible adverse reactions or unwanted effects. If you are using any other topical medications, it is advisable to speak with a healthcare professional before using products containing this plant to ensure that there are no negative interactions.

FINAL NOTE

Thank you very much for choosing this book to accompany you on your path to complete health. If you find the information, advice, or remedies I share here useful, would you do me a favor? Taking a moment to leave your review or rating (several stars would be greatly appreciated) is an incredible way to help me continue creating valuable content while also guiding others who, like you, are seeking to improve their health and well-being. Thank you so much for being part of this wellness community!

With gratitude,

Isabel

Important Note on Printing and Shipping:
All of my paperback books are printed and distributed exclusively by Amazon and its affiliated printing facilities. If you encounter any issues with print quality or delivery, please contact Amazon Customer Service directly for assistance.

As the author, I have no control over these processes, so I kindly request that your reviews focus solely on the content, remedies, or information within this work. Some readers leave negative ratings due to shipping or binding issues, unaware that these matters are, unfortunately, entirely beyond my control and ability to resolve. Thank you from the bottom of my heart for your understanding!

AUTHOR'S BOOKS

- **ACID REFLUX**. Foods, Supplements & Medicinal Plants
- **ALLERGIES**. Foods, Supplements & Herbs
- **ANXIETY**. Foods, Supplements & Herbs
- **ARTHRITIS**. Foods, Supplements & Medicinal Plants
- **CHOLESTEROL**. Foods, Supplements & Medicinal Plants
- **DIABETES**. Foods, Supplements & Herbs
- **CONSTIPATION**. Foods, Supplements & Herbs
- **FIBROMYALGIA**. Foods, Supplements & Medicinal Plants
- **GASTRITIS**. Foods, Supplements & Herbs
- **HEMORRHOIDS**. Foods, Supplements & Herbs
- **HYPERTENSION**. Foods, Supplements & Medicinal Plants
- **INSOMNIA**. Foods, Supplements & Herbs
- **MENOPAUSE**. Foods, Supplements & Medicinal Plants
- **OSTEOARTHRITIS**. Foods, Supplements & Herbs
- **SIBO**. Foods, Supplements & Medicinal Plants
- **VARICOSE VEINS**. Foods, Supplements & Herbs

Roots that Inspire: From Obstacles to New Horizons

Born in 1971 in Gáldar, Gran Canaria, Isabel grew up in an environment steeped in tradition and ancestral wisdom. Surrounded by the knowledge of her homeland, she learned from an early age to appreciate the healing power of medicinal plants, home remedies, and the importance of nutrition as foundations for nurturing both body and soul. This heritage, passed down through generations, shaped her childhood and sparked a deep passion for natural medicine–a passion that would eventually become the guiding force of her life.

The journey, however, was not without obstacles. In her youth, Isabel faced a period of profound difficulty: after her separation, she embraced the sole responsibility of raising her daughters. These were challenging times, with motherhood pushing her to her limits while simultaneously fueling her determination to persevere. Even during moments of uncertainty, she remained steadfast, drawing strength from her unwavering commitment to her values and her profound connection to natural health, which always served as her refuge and inspiration.

Rather than yielding to adversity, Isabel channeled it into a drive for learning and growth. She dedicated countless hours to studying books on medicinal plants, exploring new healing methods, and deepening her knowledge of natural remedies. Over the years, she pursued extensive training in naturopathy, nutrition, and complementary therapies, often sacrificing personal comforts to follow her passion. Her dedication not only provided for her family but also enabled her to profoundly impact the lives of those who sought her guidance. People came to trust her wisdom, turning to her for advice and support, and her efforts ignited transformations in countless lives.

A pivotal moment came in the 1990s when she made the

decision to professionalize her calling. She embarked on formal training as a naturopath and therapist specializing in alternative health practices. This step was transformative, opening new doors and broadening her ability to serve others. Her expertise, combined with her authentic desire to help, allowed her to support a growing community of people. Every story of healing and recovery deepened her sense of purpose, and she rebuilt her life around her mission to uplift others.

But Isabel's hunger for knowledge and her desire to inspire others extended beyond her immediate community. In 2017, she took a bold new step: she began to write with the aim of sharing her hard-earned experiences and knowledge on a larger scale. Her books, written in an accessible and heartfelt style, are both informative and empowering. They seamlessly blend practical advice, recipes, and natural health alternatives, inspiring readers to embrace healthier, more balanced lifestyles. Every page radiates her warmth and passion, inviting readers to find solutions for their well-being from within and aligning them to the wisdom of nature.

Today, Isabel's work resonates with countless individuals, especially those seeking to regain their health or reconnect with a more intentional way of living. Her story stands as a powerful reminder that even the greatest challenges can lead to profound purpose. Through resilience and perseverance, she has not only transformed her own life but also paved the way for others to rediscover their harmony with nature and with themselves. Her legacy serves as a celebration of living in balance with the natural world and honoring the deep, inherent connection between humanity and the Earth—a testament that obstacles can be the stepping stones to new horizons and an invitation to care for our body, mind, and planet with respect, awareness, and love.

BIBLIOGRAPHY & SCIENTIFIC STUDIES

1. "Plantas Medicinales: El Dioscórides Renovado" - Pío Font Quer

2. "The Green Pharmacy" - James A. Duke

3. "The Complete Medicinal Herbal" - Penelope Ody

4. "La Guía de las Vitaminas y Suplementos" - Sheldon Saul Hendler

5. "Herbal Medicine: Biomolecular and Clinical Aspects" - Iris F. F. Benzie y Sissi Wachtel-Galor

6. "Phytotherapy: A Quick Reference to Herbal Medicine" - Francesco Capasso

7. "Healing Herbs: A Beginner's Guide to Identifying, Foraging, and Using Medicinal Plants" - Tina Sams

8. "Plantas Medicinales y Curativas" - Jorge D. Pamplona Roger

9. "The Herbal Drugstore" - Linda B. White y Steven Foster

10. "The Encyclopedia of Medicinal Plants" - Andrew Chevallier

11. "Guía Práctica de las Vitaminas, Minerales y Suplementos Nutricionales" - Sarah Brewer

12. "A Modern Herbal" - Maud Grieve

13. "The Complete Guide to Herbal Medicines" - Charles W. Fetrow y Juan R. Avila

14. "Plantas Medicinales de Uso Tradicional en México" - Antonio Martínez y Xóchitl Hernández

15. "The New Healing Herbs: The Classic Guide to Nature's Best Medicines" - Michael Castleman

16. "Materia Médica: Plantas de Uso Terapéutico" - Mónica Koppel

17. "Herbal Remedies" - Asa Hershoff

18. "Plantas Medicinales de América Latina" - Nelson Papavero

19. "The Herbal Medicine-Maker's Handbook: A Home Manual" - James Green

20. "Manual de Fitoterapia" - J. L. Berdonces

SCIENTIFIC STUDIES
1. "Horse-chestnut seed extract for chronic venous insufficiency" - Siebert, U., Brach, M., & Lehmacher, W.

2. "Review of the horse chestnut seed extract: efficacy in the treatment of chronic venous insufficiency" - Pittler, M. H., & Ernst, E.

3. "Horse chestnut extract for venous insufficiency" - Sirtori, C. R.

4. "Diosmin: A review of its pharmacological properties and therapeutic efficacy in venous insufficiency and related disorders" - Lyseng-Williamson, K. A., & Perry, C. M.

5. "Micronized purified flavonoid fraction (MPFF): a review of its use in chronic venous insufficiency, venous ulcers and haemorrhoids" - Falanga, V., & Eaglstein, W. H.

6. "Diosmin treatment for varicose veins and venous insufficiency: A systematic review and meta-analysis" - Robertson, L., & Evans, C.

7. "The efficacy of escin in the treatment of chronic venous insufficiency: a systematic review of randomized controlled trials" - Pittler, M. H., & Ernst, E.

8. "Aescin: pharmacology, pharmacokinetics and therapeutic profile" - Sirtori, C. R.

9. "The efficacy of escin in the treatment of venous disorders: a review of the literature" - Belcaro, G., & Dugall, M.

10. "Ginkgo biloba extract in the treatment of patients with peripheral arterial occlusive disease: a controlled trial" - Peters, H., & Kieser, M.

11. "The influence of Ginkgo biloba on blood viscosity and red cell deformability in patients with peripheral arterial occlusive disease" - Jung, F., & Mrowietz, C.

12. "Ginkgo biloba extract and long-term ambulatory venous pressure: a randomized, double-blind clinical trial" - Cluzan, R., & Alliot, F.

13. "Hesperidin: Therapeutic Potential in Venous Insufficiency and Beyond" - Garg, A., & Garg, S.

14. "Hesperidin in the treatment of chronic venous insufficiency" - Mariani, P., & Mariani, F.

15. "Effect of hesperidin on capillary permeability" - Faggiotto, A., & Rossato, P.

16. "Niacin and vascular function: a review of evidence-based mechanisms" - Kamanna, V. S., & Kashyap, M. L.

17. "Niacin: an old drug with a new twist" - Ganji, S. H., & Kamanna, V. S.

18. "The role of nicotinic acid in the management of dyslipidemia" - McKenney, J. M., & Proctor, J. D.

19. "Effects of rutin and flavonoids on venous insufficiency: a systematic review" - Martínez, M. J., & Vicente, M.

20. "Rutin in venous disease: a review" - Belcaro, G., & Cesarone, M. R.

21. "Rutosides as a treatment for chronic venous insufficiency: a meta-analysis of randomized controlled trials" - Martínez-Zapata, M. J., & Moreno, R. M.

22. "Vitamin C and vascular health" - Carr, A. C., & Frei, B.

23. "The role of vitamin C in prevention and treatment of venous disease" - Padayatty, S. J., & Levine, M.

24. "Vitamin C supplementation reduces the occurrence of complex regional pain syndrome in foot and ankle surgery" - Zollinger, P. E., & Tuinebreijer, W. E.

25. "Vitamin E and cardiovascular health: the anti-inflammatory perspective" - Devaraj, S., & Jialal, I.

26. "The role of vitamin E in the prevention of atherosclerosis and chronic venous insufficiency" - Riccioni, G., & Bucciarelli, T.

27. "Vitamin E supplementation in cardiovascular disease prevention: a meta-analysis" - Myung, S. K., & Ju, W.

28. "Equisetum arvense in the treatment of venous insufficiency: a review" - Vieira, M. R., & Silva, M. P.

29. "The use of Equisetum arvense (horsetail) in the treatment of venous disorders" - Blumenthal, M., & Goldberg, A.

30. "Cola de caballo: propiedades y aplicaciones en la insuficiencia venosa" - García, M. J

31. "Hamamelis extract in the treatment of chronic venous insufficiency: a review" - Wananukul, S., & Chatproedprai, S.

32. "The role of witch hazel in vascular health and venous insufficiency" - Wendt, M., & Müller, T.

33. "Hamamelis extract for the treatment of varicose veins: a systematic review" - Greeske, K., & Pohlmann, B.

34. "Ginger (Zingiber officinale) in the treatment of vascular disorders: a review" - Ali, B. H., & Blunden, G.

35. "The effects of ginger on human health: a comprehensive review" - Mashhadi, N. S., & Ghiasvand, R.

36. "Ginger and its effect on blood circulation and vascular health" - Thomson, M., & Al-Qattan, K. K.

37. "Malva sylvestris: A review of its traditional uses, phytochemistry, and pharmacological properties" - Barros, L., & Carvalho, A. M.

38. "The potential of Malva sylvestris in the treatment of venous insufficiency" - Aktay, G., & Deliorman, D.

39. "Malva extracts for vascular health: a review" - Conforti, F., & Menichini, F.

40. "Ruscus aculeatus extract in the treatment of chronic venous insufficiency: a meta-analysis" - Pittler, M. H., & Ernst, E.

41. "The efficacy of Ruscus in the management of venous disorders:

a review" - Belcaro, G., & Cesarone, M. R.

42. "Ruscus aculeatus in venous insufficiency: a systematic review" - Vanscheidt, W., & Rabe, E.

43. "Vitis vinifera (red vine leaf) extract in the treatment of chronic venous insufficiency: a systematic review" - Diehm, C., & Trampisch, H. J.

44. "The role of red vine leaf extract in vascular health" - Cesarone, M. R., & Belcaro, G.

45. "Clinical efficacy of red vine leaf extract in chronic venous insufficiency: a meta-analysis" - Belcaro, G., & Nicolaides, A. N.

www.ingramcontent.com/pod-product-compliance
Lightning Source LLC
Chambersburg PA
CBHW061046250726
48653CB00001B/275